Fast Facts

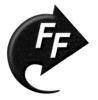

Fast Facts:
Skin Cancer

Second edition

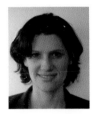

Karen L Agnew MBChB FRACP
Consultant Dermatologist
Auckland City and Starship Children's Hospitals
Auckland, New Zealand

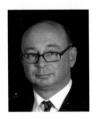

Christopher B Bunker MA MD FRCP
Consultant Dermatologist
University College and Chelsea and Westminster Hospitals,
and Professor of Dermatology
University College and Imperial College
London, UK

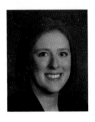

Sarah T Arron MD PhD
Assistant Professor of Dermatology
Director, High Risk Skin Cancer Program
Chief of Mohs Micrographic Surgery, San Francisco
Veterans Administration Medical Center
University of California, San Francisco
CA, USA

Declaration of Independence
This book is as balanced and as practical as we can make it.
Ideas for improvement are always welcome: feedback@fastfacts.com

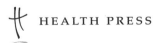

HEALTH PRESS

Fast Facts: Skin Cancer
First published August 2005; reprinted 2007
Second edition 2013; reprinted June 2015 (with revisions, pages 80–1)

Text © 2013 Karen L Agnew, Christopher B Bunker, Sarah T Arron
© 2013 in this edition Health Press Limited
Health Press Limited, Elizabeth House, Queen Street, Abingdon,
Oxford OX14 3LN, UK
Tel: +44 (0)1235 523233
Fax: +44 (0)1235 523238

Book orders can be placed by telephone or via the website.
For regional distributors or to order via the website, please go to:
fastfacts.com

For telephone orders, please call +44 1752 202301 (UK, Europe and Asia–Pacific),
1 800 247 6553 (USA, toll free) or +1 419 281 1802 (Americas).

Fast Facts is a trademark of Health Press Limited.

The photographs in this book are reproduced courtesy of Medical Illustration UK
Ltd, Chelsea and Westminster Hospital, London, UK, and Aleks Itkin MD, Scripps
Clinic, La Jolla, CA, USA.

The publisher and the authors have made every effort to ensure the accuracy of this
book, but cannot accept responsibility for any errors or omissions.

For all drugs, please consult the product labeling approved in your country for
prescribing information.

A CIP record for this title is available from the British Library.

ISBN 978-1-908541-39-0

Agnew, K (Karen)
Fast Facts: Skin Cancer/
Karen L Agnew, Christopher B Bunker, Sarah T Arron

Medical illustrations by Annamaria Dutto, Withernsea, UK.
Typesetting and page layout by Zed, Oxford, UK.
Printed by Charlesworth Press, Wakefield, UK.

Glossary

Actinic keratosis (solar keratosis): a sun-induced precancerous cutaneous lesion, presenting as a scaly patch or plaque, comprising atypical keratinocytes microscopically

5-ALA: 5-aminolevulinic acid – a naturally occurring substance in the human body that is converted to protoporphyrin IX, a photosensitizer, especially in actively growing cells; often present in precancers or cancers

Basal cell carcinoma (BCC): a low-grade skin cancer; the most common human malignancy, composed microscopically of basaloid cells, which are locally invasive and rarely metastasize

Bowen's disease: a scaly erythematous plaque that is a type of in situ squamous cell carcinoma

Breslow thickness: cutaneous melanoma thickness, measured histologically from the top of the viable epidermis (granular layer) to the deepest tumor cell in the skin; an important prognostic indicator

Chondrodermatitis nodularis helicis: a small, benign but painful papule on the helix of the ear caused by inflammation of the ear cartilage

Clark's level of invasion: a grading system for the level of invasion of primary cutaneous melanoma. Like Breslow thickness, it correlates with risk of metastasis, with a worse prognosis for the higher levels:

- Level I is confined to the epidermis
- Level II extends to the papillary dermis past the basement membrane
- Level III fills the papillary dermis and compresses the reticular dermis
- Level IV invades the reticular dermis
- Level V involves subcutaneous tissue

Cryosurgery: a dermatologic treatment in which a very cold substance or cryogen (usually liquid nitrogen) is applied to the skin to freeze cutaneous lesions and cause controlled necrosis

Dermascope/dermatoscope: a handheld magnifying instrument that assists with the examination of cutaneous lesions

Epidermolysis bullosa dystrophica: an inherited blistering disease, characterized by atrophy of blistered areas, severe scarring and nail changes that occur after separation of the epidermis

Erythema ab igne: a red-brown hyperpigmentation of the skin caused by chronic local exposure to heat

Erythroplasia of Queyrat: squamous cell carcinoma in situ of unkeratinized genital epithelium, i.e. uncircumcised men

Gorlin's syndrome: an inherited disease in which a mutated gene (*PTCH1*) predisposes to development of tens to hundreds of BCC and to certain other developmental anomalies (also known as basal cell nevus syndrome and nevoid basal cell carcinoma syndrome)

Hedgehog signaling pathway: a cascade of signaling molecules that influence embryologic development and later cell division, in which mutations can lead to BCC and other malignancies

HPV: human papillomavirus, responsible for warts; only certain subtypes are related to the development of cancer

Hyperkeratosis: thickening of the outer layer of skin

In situ: in place – a cancer that has not spread to invade neighboring tissues

Keratinocyte: a cell of the epidermis characterized by keratin production

Keratoacanthoma: a rapidly growing epidermal tumor comprising well-differentiated atypical keratinocytes; the tumor usually regresses spontaneously; more aggressive forms are often difficult to differentiate from squamous cell carcinoma. It is probably best regarded as a variant of squamous carcinoma

Lentigo (plural: lentigines): a dark spot with more pigment cells than normal skin; a sign of sun damage but lacking malignant potential

Lentigo maligna (Hutchinson's melanotic freckle): an irregularly pigmented macule most commonly found on the face and/or neck of older people representing in situ melanoma with the potential to progress into invasive malignant melanoma (lentigo maligna melanoma)

MAL: methyl aminolevulinate – used as a photosensitizer in photodynamic therapy

Mammillated: having nipple-like projections

Melanocyte: a melanin-producing cell situated in the basal layer of the epidermis; the normal counterpart of a melanoma cell

Melanoma: a cutaneous tumor with strong metastatic potential, comprising malignant melanocytes

Mohs micrographic surgery: a procedure in which a cutaneous neoplasm is excised and the margins frozen-sectioned and assessed histologically in stages as the tumor is removed; the wound is only repaired when there is histological confirmation of complete excision

Nevomelanocyte: precursor of a melanocytic nevus cell derived from either epidermal melanoblasts or dermal Schwann cells

Nevus: developmental abnormality. A melanocytic nevus (commonly a mole); a cluster of benign pigment cells that usually appear in the first decades of life ('bathing trunk' nevi are congenital lesions that cover a large area of the body)

Parakeratosis: retention of nuclei in the upper layers of the epidermis

Photodynamic therapy (PDT): a treatment in which a photosensitizer such as 5-ALA or MAL is applied to the tissue and then activated by a source of visible light, resulting in cell destruction

Punch biopsy: a small skin specimen for histological assessment obtained by using a circular blade attached to a handle

PUVA: administration of psoralen (a phototoxic drug), which acts as a skin sensitizer, followed by exposure to ultraviolet A (UVA) light; used to treat psoriasis, vitiligo and other skin diseases

Seborrheic keratosis: a benign pigmented, often papillomatous, cutaneous lesion generally seen in older individuals; also called stucco keratosis

Squamous cell carcinoma (SCC): a malignant cutaneous neoplasm, derived from keratinocytes, that usually presents as an enlarging nodule on sun-exposed sites; these tumors have metastatic potential

Sunburn cells: keratinocytes undergoing apoptosis as a result of UV irradiation

Sun protection factor (SPF): a number that quantifies the degree of protection given by a sunscreen from the erythemogenic wavelengths (primarily UVB). The SPF value is obtained by dividing the exposure time required to develop barely detectable erythema (sunburn) for sunscreen-protected skin by that for unprotected skin

UPF: ultraviolet protection factor; the degree of UV protectiveness of a fabric, calculated by measuring the transmission of UVA and UVB through given fabrics with a spectrophotometer. Fabrics with a tight weave, a dark color and a heavy weight have a higher UPF (e.g. denim=1700) and are more protective

UV: ultraviolet; the portion of sunlight energy responsible for sunburn, tanning and cancer

Xeroderma pigmentosum: a rare autosomal-recessive disorder of defective DNA repair characterized by more than a thousandfold risk of UV-induced skin cancer

Introduction

Skin cancer is the most common human cancer worldwide, and the incidence continues to increase. However, most skin cancers are preventable and treatable. It is of crucial importance for all of us to understand how we can prevent, diagnose and treat these common cancers. *Fast Facts: Skin Cancer* provides essential information that will help healthcare professionals, medical students and the public to understand this important and rapidly evolving area of medicine.

There are three main types of skin cancer: malignant melanoma and the two non-melanoma skin cancers, basal cell carcinoma (BCC) and squamous cell carcinoma (SCC). Most skin malignancies are curable if they are diagnosed early enough, but both melanoma, in particular, and SCC can kill.

Theoretically, skin cancer can be prevented by educating people about recreational habits, clothing, sunscreens and sunbeds (primary prevention), but this approach could take a generation or more before it has a sizeable effect. Meanwhile, emerging evidence surrounding the role of vitamin D means that physicians need to consider supplementation for individuals adhering to strict sun avoidance practices.

When skin cancer does occur, early recognition and specialist referral saves lives. Serious morbidity and mortality can be prevented or reduced by educating patients and physicians alike, so that at-risk individuals and early lesions are identified with accuracy. There are nine tumors on the cover of this book, and three of them are malignant cancers – can you identify them? This book will show you how.

Surgery is usually the treatment of choice for skin cancer, although there are other options. Although relatively simple surgery suffices for most cancers in most patients, some require multidisciplinary input from a dermatologist, surgeon, pathologist, radiotherapist or radiation oncologist, and medical oncologist. Mohs micrographic surgery has resulted in significantly improved cure rates for selected skin cancers, particularly the non-melanoma skin cancers BCC and SCC. Yet, despite recent advances in the treatment of disseminated disease, our methods remain inaccurate and mortality of metastatic skin cancer is high.

In this second edition of *Fast Facts: Skin Cancer* we present updated facts about the epidemiology and causation of skin cancer, alongside a commonsense approach to identification and management. Our aim is to provide an evidence-based, practical resource that will answer common questions, and reflect the national and international consensus guidelines that are constantly evolving. It will assist practice, education, training, audit and research.

Fast Facts: Skin Cancer is written by dermatologists to provide you with the information that your dermatologist wants you to know. We have designed an easy-to-read, fact-filled and practical primer to skin cancer. Whether you are a physician, nurse, medical student or other healthcare professional, or an interested patient or curious layman, this book is for you. Read on and join the effort to prevent and treat skin cancer!

Acknowledgment: We would like to thank Dr Barbara A Gilchrest, Professor of Dermatology, Boston University School of Medicine, for her contribution to the first edition of this handbook.

Basal cell carcinoma

Basal cell carcinoma (BCC) is the most common malignant neoplasm in white individuals. Its incidence has increased in recent decades: the highest rates are in Australia, where it affects over 2% of men. In the UK, USA, Australia and New Zealand these basic data are still not collected centrally and estimates vary. Extrapolated data reported in a recent paper suggest that, in 2010, approximately 200 000 patients were treated surgically for 247 000 BCCs in the UK.

The tumor most commonly arises on the head and neck (Figure 1.1) and, overall, the incidence is higher in men than in women.

Risk factors. The risk of BCC is increased in those who:
- had episodes of severe childhood sunburn
- have red hair
- tan poorly.

The association with sunlight is not well understood. Cumulative ultraviolet (UV) radiation was thought to be the most important risk factor. However, exposure to the sun during childhood and

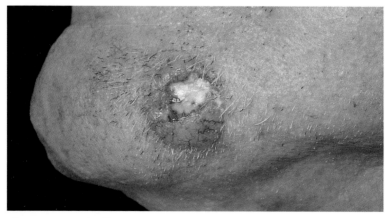

Figure 1.1 Basal cell carcinoma most commonly arises on the head and neck.

adolescence – particularly intense intermittent exposure –may be of greater importance in the development of BCC than previously thought.

Other risk factors for BCC include:

- North European ancestry
- a positive family history
- immunosuppression
- exposure to arsenic
- previous radiotherapy.

BCC can develop in a sebaceous nevus (Figure 1.2). It is also associated with a number of conditions, including albinism, xeroderma pigmentosum (a rare autosomal-recessive disorder that affects DNA repair), nevoid BCC syndrome (Gorlin's syndrome) and HIV infection.

Table 1.1 summarizes the risk factors for BCC compared with squamous cell carcinoma (SCC) and melanoma.

Squamous cell carcinoma

Cutaneous SCC is the second most common skin cancer in white individuals; SCC represents roughly 20% of all non-melanoma skin carcinomas. The incidence of non-melanoma skin cancer (BCC and SCC together) is approximately 18–20-fold greater than that of melanoma.

SCC is most commonly seen in the elderly and is three times more common in men than women. The incidence is rising, and is highest

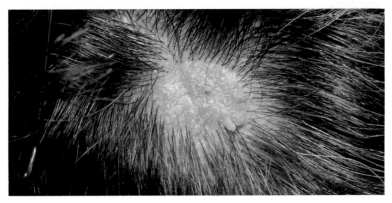

Figure 1.2 Sebaceous nevus on scalp – basal cell carcinoma and squamous cell carcinoma can develop from this type of birthmark.

TABLE 1.1

Risk factors for skin cancer

	Basal cell carcinoma	Squamous cell carcinoma	Melanoma
Sex	Male > female	Male > female	Male > female
Relationship to sun exposure	Childhood; intermittent	Chronic	Childhood; intermittent
Sunburn history	Severe sunburn in childhood	Episode of severe sunburn	Episode of severe sunburn
Tanning ability	Non-tanners	Non-tanners	Non-tanners
Skin color	Fair skin/freckles	Fair skin/freckles	Fair skin/ freckles
Hair color	Red	Red/blond	Red/blond
Eye color	Light eye color	Light eye color	Blue
Precursor lesions	Actinic keratosis	Actinic keratosis	Nevi

in countries with high sun exposure. Non-melanoma skin cancer morbidity and mortality statistics are not registered in the UK, USA, New Zealand or Australia. The American Cancer Society estimates that 3.5 million cases of non-melanoma skin cancer were diagnosed in 2006. In Australia, the total number of non-melanoma skin cancer treatments rose to 767 347 in 2010, and it has been suggested that UK figures are likely to be similar.

Lesions occur on sun-exposed sites, predominantly the head and neck (Figure 1.3).

Risk factors. UV radiation is the strongest etiologic factor. In particular, sun exposure, both recent and cumulative, is implicated in SCC development. This malignancy is more common in fair-skinned individuals with red or blond hair (see Table 1.1).

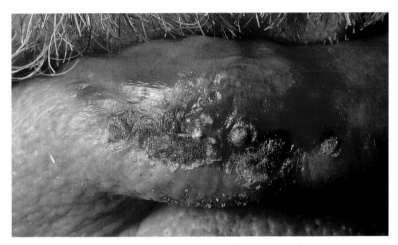

Figure 1.3 Squamous cell carcinoma on the lip – these lesions predominantly occur on sun-exposed sites, particularly the head and neck.

The acquired risk factors for SCC include:
- a history of severe sunburn
- sunbed use
- 200+ treatments with psoralen and UVA phototherapy (PUVA) (e.g. for psoriasis)
- smoking
- chronic immunosuppression (as occurs with alcoholism, HIV infection, chronic lymphatic leukemia and organ transplantation).

Much of the research identifying the association between immunosuppression and SCC has been performed in the organ transplant population. The risk of developing SCC is increased in organ transplant recipients, and the ratio of BCC to SCC incidence is reversed in this population.

Other predisposing factors for SCC include previous exposure to polycyclic hydrocarbons or radiation (Figure 1.4), exposure to arsenic, and infection with the human papillomavirus (HPV). Further genetic risk factors include conditions with *P53* (also known as *TP53*) gene mutation, xeroderma pigmentosum and albinism.

In addition, invasive SCC is recognized to develop from actinic keratosis and in situ SCC, as well as at sites of chronic injury, such as ulceration, infection, scars and epidermolysis bullosa

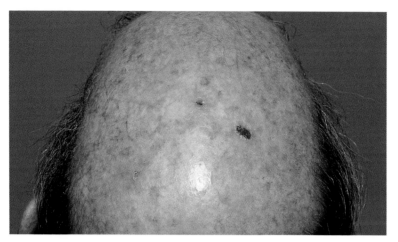

Figure 1.4 Radiotherapy-damaged scalp on which a squamous cell carcinoma subsequently developed.

dystrophica (a condition characterized by atrophy of blistered areas and severe scarring).

Melanoma

The incidence of melanoma is increasing faster than that of any other human cancer. It primarily affects white-skinned people, in whom the incidence increases with age and is inversely related to the latitude of residence. Melanoma occurs more commonly in men, and mortality is higher in men, particularly in those aged over 50. It is most commonly found on the faces or backs of white men and the limbs of white women (Figure 1.5).

Plantar and subungual melanomas are very rare, but when melanoma develops at these sites it is seen most often in black populations and people from South East Asia and the Indian subcontinent.

Internationally, the incidence of melanoma varies: it is highest in New Zealand and Australia, where melanoma is the fourth most common cancer. In Australia, 1 in 14 men and 1 in 23 women are expected to develop melanoma in their lifetime. The highest rates of melanoma are found in New Zealand, where there are approximately 51 melanomas per 100 000 people per year. The UK incidence is

13

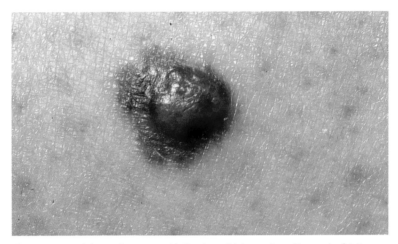

Figure 1.5 Nodular melanoma, with Breslow thickness (see Glossary) of 1.8 mm.

26.6 per 100 000 people per year (12 800 cases in 2010 [Cancer Research UK statistics]). In the USA, the incidence is significantly lower in non-white ethnic groups, ranging from 1 per 100 000 per year in black Americans and Asian Americans to 4 per 100 000 per year in American Indians and Hispanics. Fortunately, there is evidence that survival rates improve as the proportion of 'thin' melanoma (≤ 0.75 mm) being diagnosed increases. In New South Wales, Australia, the overall 5-year survival rate for melanoma was 50% in 1980, whereas in 2000 it had improved to 85%.

Risk factors. The development of superficial spreading and nodular melanoma correlates more with exposure to intermittent intense sunlight than with chronic UV radiation. The risk of melanoma (see Table 1.1) is largely genetically determined and increases in people with:
- fair complexion
- freckles
- blue eyes
- red or blond hair.
  Other predisposing factors include:
- an increased number of normal (Figure 1.6) or atypical nevi
- a history of sunburn, particularly before 15 years of age

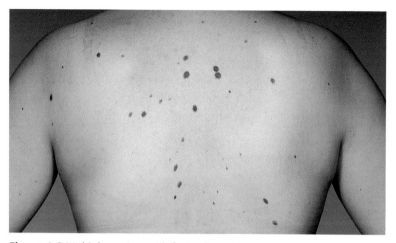

Figure 1.6 Multiple nevi – a risk factor for melanoma.

- an inability to tan
- sunbed use.

A positive family history is also a risk factor, predominantly as a consequence of predisposing family traits. The term familial malignant melanoma is used when two or more first-degree relatives develop melanoma. These individuals tend to develop multiple melanomas, primarily occurring at a lower stage (see Table 3.6, page 66); the age at onset is lower than in the general population. Familial malignant melanoma accounts for 5–12% of all melanomas; only a small subset of affected individuals are likely to have an inherited melanoma susceptibility gene mutation. Predisposing genes have been identified, one of which is also identified with pancreatic cancer (this is covered briefly in Chapter 2).

Other risk factors for malignant melanoma include:
- iatrogenic immunosuppression
- PUVA treatment (e.g. for psoriasis)
- xeroderma pigmentosum
- HIV infection
- atypical nevus syndrome (see page 39).

Malignant melanoma can develop from congenital or acquired melanocytic nevi. In patients with congenital melanocytic nevi (CMN), the lifetime risk of melanoma is not well established; the most recent

15

systematic review calculates a 0.7% overall risk of melanoma developing in these individuals. This risk strongly depends on CMN size; melanoma arising from small- to medium-sized CMN is rare. The risk is highest in CMN with diameter greater than 40 cm; melanoma develops in 2.5–5% of giant 'bathing trunk' lesions – congenital lesions that cover large areas of the body.

Key points – epidemiology

- Deaths from skin cancer continue to rise.
- Ultraviolet radiation is the most important risk factor.
- Early diagnosis saves lives.

Key references

Australian Cancer Network Melanoma Guidelines Revision Working Party. *Clinical Practice Guidelines for the Management of Melanoma in Australia and New Zealand.* Wellington: Cancer Council Australia and Australian Cancer Network, Sydney and New Zealand Guidelines Group, 2008. Available at www.nhmrc.gov.au/_files_nhmrc/publications/attachments/cp111.pdf, last accessed 19 August 2013.

Bagheri MM, Safai B. Cutaneous malignancies of keratinocytic origin. *Clin Dermatol* 2001;19:244–52.

Bunker CB, Gotch F. AIDS and the skin. In: Burns T, Breathnach S, Cox N, Griffiths C, eds. *Rook's Textbook of Dermatology*, 7th edn. Oxford: Blackwell Science, 2004: 26.1–26.41.

Cancer Research UK. Skin cancer statistics. Available at www.cancerresearchuk.org/cancer-info/cancerstats/types/skin, last accessed 19 August 2013.

Fransen M, Karahalios A, Sharma N et al. Non-melanoma skin cancer in Australia. *Med J Aust* 2012;197: 565–8.

Goldstein AM, Tucker MA. Genetic epidemiology of cutaneous melanoma: a global perspective. *Arch Dermatol* 2001;137:1493–6.

Howlader N, Noone AM, Krapcho M et al., eds. *SEER Cancer Statistics Review, 1975–2009 (Vintage 2009 Populations)*. Bethesda: National Cancer Institute. http://seer.cancer.gov/csr/1975_2009_pops09, based on November 2011 SEER data submission, posted to the SEER website, April 2012.

Krengel S, Hauschild A, Schafer T. Melanoma risk in congenital melanocytic naevi: a systematic review. *Br J Dermatol* 2006;155: 1–8.

Leonardi-Bee J, Ellison T, Bath-Hextall F. Smoking and the risk of nonmelanoma skin cancer: systematic review and meta-analysis. *Arch Dermatol* 2012;148:939–46.

Levell NJ, Igali L, Wright KA, Greenberg DC. Basal cell carcinoma epidemiology in the UK: the elephant in the room. *Clin Exp Dermatol* 2013;38:367–9.

Roest MAB, Keane FM, Agnew K et al. Multiple squamous skin carcinomas following excess sunbed use. *J R Soc Med* 2001;94:636–7.

Shah KN. The risk of melanoma and neurocutaneous melanosis associated with congenital melanocytic nevi. *Semin Cutan Med Surg* 2010;29: 159–64.

Sinclair R. Nonmelanoma skin cancer in Australia (Editorial). *Br J Dermatol* 2013;168:1–2.

Stern RS. PUVA follow up study. The risk of melanoma in association with long-term exposure to PUVA. *J Am Acad Dermatol* 2001;44: 755–61.

Malignancy

Integrity of the genome is critical to life. Even one miscoded or incorrectly expressed protein can have catastrophic results. In higher organisms such as man, disturbing the exquisite balance between growth and differentiation of cells in a way that leads to cancer is a relatively common and sometimes lethal error.

In the skin, it is necessary for cells to divide throughout life. The outer layer is continuously shed and must be replaced by terminally differentiating cells generated from the layers just below. If cell division and differentiation fail, infection and electrolyte loss can rapidly lead to death. Yet too much cell division, coupled with impaired differentiation, constitutes a malignant tumor. The excess cells can also migrate elsewhere (metastasis), divide in other parts of the body and severely impair organ function.

Oncogenes. Many decades ago, researchers discovered that infection with certain viruses caused malignant tumors in animals. They then found that specific viral genes, termed oncogenes or cancer-causing genes, encoded proteins that caused uncontrolled growth of infected cells. Normal mammalian cells were found to contain very similar or identical genes that functioned or 'turned on' proteins in response to specific signals to stimulate cell division; mutated gene products (proteins) could be permanently 'turned on', like the viral oncogene products, leading to continuous inappropriate cell division or cancer. The normal unmutated versions of such genes are now termed proto-oncogenes, implying that they can be converted to oncogenes. Common examples belong to the RAS family of proto-oncogenes. Mutations in such genes are usually dominant (that is, abnormal proliferation occurs if one of the two copies of the gene in a cell is mutated).

Tumor suppressor genes. A second group of genes that contribute to cancer was discovered in children at high risk of retinoblastoma.

Affected children often lost both eyes to these malignant retinal growths and, if they survived, they often died of a third malignancy in another organ. These children were found to have a mutation in one copy of the retinoblastoma gene of which the protein product (pRb) served as a critical 'brake' on cell growth, especially in certain cell types. If the second normal copy of the gene was inactivated for any reason, the affected cells would begin to divide uncontrollably. Further research has revealed many such tumor suppressor genes and cancer-prone syndromes in which one gene copy is abnormal from birth (or, in most cases, from conception) and a later random mutation of the second copy leads to malignancy. In families strongly predisposed to dysplastic nevi and melanoma, the inherited mutation is usually in the CDKN2A gene that encodes two tumor suppressor proteins, p16INK4a and p14ARF. Mutations in this gene also predispose family members to other malignancies, notably pancreatic carcinoma.

Perhaps the best known tumor suppressor gene is P53 (also known as TP53), which encodes p53 'the guardian of the genome': a transcription factor and DNA-repair protein that is dysfunctional in half of all human malignancies. It is now clear that loss of function of the tumor suppressor gene is extremely common in spontaneous malignancies, despite the requirement for both copies of the gene to be compromised, a statistically rare event. This is strong testimony to the important role of tumor suppressor proteins in modulating normal cell growth.

Carcinogens. Cancer develops as a result of cumulative DNA damage, most often because of a combination of carcinogen exposure and genetic vulnerability. Ultraviolet (UV) radiation (sun exposure) is the most important contributory factor for skin cancer, but in some individuals exposure to other carcinogens, such as cigarette smoke or chewing tobacco, arsenic or therapeutic irradiation, may also contribute.

A classic early example of skin cancer developing as a consequence of carcinogen exposure was the development of otherwise rare scrotal cancers in chimney sweeps in England. The cancers were caused by exposure of this vulnerable area of skin to the chemicals present in soot, which penetrated clothes.

Effect of age. The incidence of all skin cancers rises exponentially with age. In part, this is because cumulative mutations are acquired over time. Vulnerability to new damage also appears to increase with age, in part because of decreased production of DNA-repair proteins.

Photocarcinogenesis

The role of UV radiation is twofold:

- damage to the DNA, causing mutations in the genes that regulate cell growth, including proto-oncogenes and tumor suppressor genes
- an immunosuppressive effect on the skin.

UVB radiation is more photocarcinogenic than UVA, photon for photon, but UVA is far more abundant in sunlight. It is likely that both contribute to the development of skin cancer.

When UV photons are absorbed by DNA, photoproducts or distorted linkages form. The most common is the dimeric fusion product of two adjacent DNA pyrimidine bases (cytosine [C] or thymine [T]) (Figure 2.1). The predominant photoproduct, accounting for up to 85% of DNA lesions after UV radiation, is the cyclobutane pyrimidine dimer. If not properly repaired, the photoproduct can lead to a point mutation in the DNA because DNA polymerase is unable to interpret the altered bases and inserts the wrong 'partner' in the new complementary DNA strand that it synthesizes (Figure 2.2). Fortunately, before DNA synthesis occurs, the photoproducts are usually repaired by nucleotide excision repair enzymes, which avert tumor formation. However, there is evidence that this capacity to repair DNA declines with age, leading to an increased risk of unrepaired mutations.

In normal circumstances, lymphocytes appear capable of destroying malignant cells by recognizing the new proteins (antigens) they often express on their surface. However, UV radiation induces cutaneous immunosuppression, which favors tumor survival. The mechanism of UV-induced immunosuppression, which has been extensively studied in mice, is not completely understood. However, sunlight causes cells to release immunosuppressive chemicals or cytokines and alters the

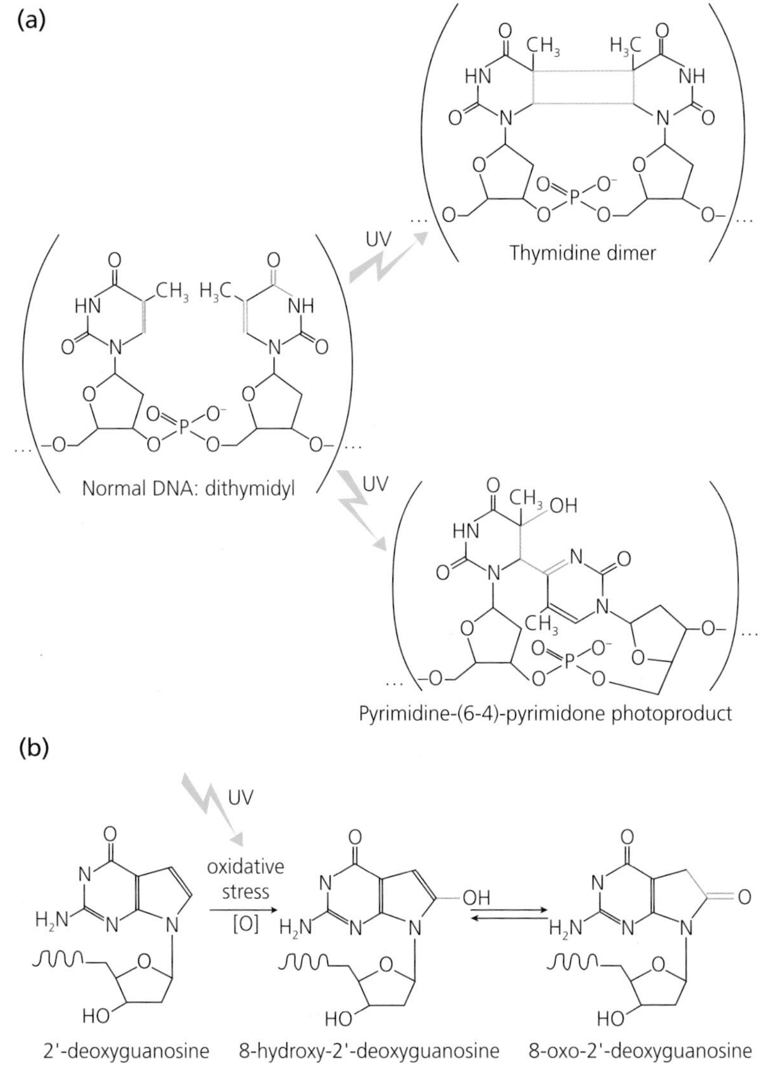

Figure 2.1 Ultraviolet (UV)-induced DNA damage. (a) UV photons may be absorbed directly by DNA, leading to new covalent bonds between adjacent pyrimidines. Both cyclobutane pyrimidine dimers (more common) and (6-4)-pyrimidine–pyrimidone photoproducts may be formed. (b) Both UVB and UVA can also damage DNA by producing free radicals that, in turn, oxidize DNA bases, usually guanine. If unrepaired, either type of damage can lead to a DNA point mutation.

21

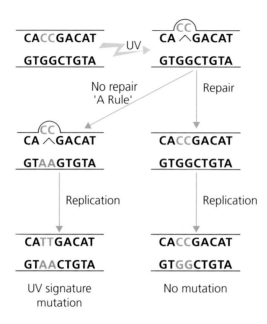

Figure 2.2 Ultraviolet (UV) radiation is the only carcinogen to produce pyrimidine photoproducts (distorted pyrimidine bases; see Figure 2.1). When unable to 'read' bases properly during DNA replication, DNA polymerase uses the 'A rule' and places adenosine (A) opposite the distorted unreadable base(s). The most characteristic UV signature mutation is C→T, which occurs only where a cytosine (C) lies next to a thymine (T) or another cystosine. In the arbitrary gene sequence above an unrepaired UV-induced CC dimer results in AA on the new complementary strand. This, in turn, dictates TT rather than CC during the next round of DNA replication, producing a UV signature mutation. Other non-UV carcinogens and even normal cellular metabolism can cause damage to other DNA bases, especially guanine (G). A damaged G paired with an A will give rise to a G→T mutation, but this is not a UV signature mutation.

antigen-presenting function of Langerhans cells. Sunlight may also play a role in the generation of suppressor rather than helper T lymphocytes, which dampens the immune response to 'foreign' cells.

Genetic predisposition

Most (perhaps all) tumors result from DNA mutations in the genes responsible for regulating cellular growth or DNA repair. Multiple genetic lesions in a single cell are usually required before its unregulated growth gives rise to a solid tumor.

There are a number of recognized genetic mutations associated with cutaneous malignancies.

P53 is a tumor suppressor gene (as discussed on pages 18–19) that influences many cellular functions, including cell cycle arrest, programmed cell death, cellular differentiation and DNA repair. It is also a transcription factor and, as such, can increase or decrease the production of other gene products. The encoded p53 phosphoprotein recognizes DNA injury and arrests cell division to provide time for DNA repair; if the DNA damage is severe, p53 induces cell apoptosis. UV-induced *P53* gene mutations are seen in nearly all squamous cell carcinomas (SCCs) and approximately 50% of basal cell carcinomas (BCCs). *P53* mutations are also common in sun-damaged skin, premalignant actinic keratoses and Bowen's disease. This suggests that loss of p53 function occurs early in the stepwise progression from a completely normal epidermal cell to a frankly malignant one, probably because the loss of p53 function makes it easier for other mutations to accumulate in cells.

Xeroderma pigmentosum. Patients with this rare disease have a mutation in one of the genes encoding proteins involved in nucleotide excision repair, which is involved in the removal of UV-induced DNA damage. When DNA damage in growth-regulating genes is not repaired, tumors can arise. The initial clinical presentation is exaggerated sunburn within the first 2 years of life. Children then develop pigmented macules, atrophy and scarring on sun-exposed sites. The predominant cutaneous malignancies are BCC and SCC, although the incidence of melanoma is significantly increased in these children. This can only be prevented by early diagnosis and complete protection from the sun, starting in infancy.

PTCH1. The patched 1 gene (*PTCH1*) is another tumor suppressor gene. It has a central role in the so-called hedgehog signaling pathway that stimulates growth. In autosomal-dominant nevoid BCC syndrome (Gorlin's syndrome), one copy of *PTCH1* is mutated and inactive in all body cells. As for pRb and retinoblastoma discussed previously, if the second gene copy is lost in a single cell the cell begins to divide excessively and a tumor develops. Patients with Gorlin's syndrome often have hundreds of BCCs that start to develop in adolescence. *PTCH1* mutations are also common in sporadic BCC.

RAS family. The RAS family of proto-oncogenes encode G proteins involved in growth-factor signaling. Mutations in RAS genes have been found in cutaneous melanoma, SCC and actinic keratosis.

CDKN2A. Inherited *CDKN2A* mutations have been identified in some relatives of people who have a genetic predisposition for melanoma. Many sporadic melanomas are also found to have mutations or loss of expression of this tumor suppressor gene, known to act in the same signaling pathway as pRb.

MC1R. Another genetic predisposition to skin cancer involves *MC1R*, which encodes melanocortin-1 receptor, the cell-surface receptor for α-melanocyte-stimulating hormone (α-MSH). Although originally named for their roles in stimulating pigment production in skin and hair, these proteins are now also known to influence immune function and possibly even DNA repair. Variants of the normal *MC1R* gene sequence are common in humans, and some less active variants have been strongly linked to fair freckled skin and red or blond hair, as well as to a high risk of skin cancer, including melanoma. The receptor encoded by these variants is not considered a mutant, but it signals far less well than the normal receptor after binding α-MSH, and is likely to contribute directly to the predisposition for cancer, at the very least by compromising protective melanin production. Such variations among key proteins still considered to be within the 'normal' range almost certainly contribute to cancer predisposition in the skin and indeed in all organ systems as observed in the general population.

Other predisposing factors

In addition to the specific gene mutations described above, viral infections have been shown to affect the pathogenesis of SCC. Particular strains of human papillomavirus (HPV) have high oncogenic potential and have been implicated in the development of in situ and invasive SCC of the anogenital region and nail unit. Here, viral DNA is incorporated into the host genome, influencing cell differentiation and growth. Viral genes that inactivate *P53* have been studied in detail.

Immunocompromised individuals – for example, organ transplant recipients or those with HIV infection – have an increased risk of non-melanoma skin cancer. It is presumed that dysplastic keratinocytes are not identified or are not eradicated effectively by immune surveillance, and malignancies are more likely to develop.

Relationship to pattern of ultraviolet exposure

Cutaneous melanoma arises from epidermal melanocytes, whereas SCC and BCC develop from keratinocytes. Although UV radiation plays a major role in all three malignancies, the patterns of UV exposure associated with the malignancies differ. Melanoma is associated with intense intermittent exposure to sunlight, and it most commonly develops on sites of the body that receive UV intermittently. In contrast, SCC is associated with chronic cumulative sun exposure. This type of malignancy tends to occur in people with substantial daily sun exposure, such as farmers or sailors, and in habitually maximally sun-exposed sites.

The reason for these differences is unknown, but recent insights into how cells respond to UV radiation allow for speculation. The melanocytes produce melanin and distribute it to surrounding keratinocytes. Melanin is hence able to absorb UV photons that might otherwise damage DNA or cell membranes and is photoprotective. When skin is irradiated with sunlight, melanin production increases, as does the capacity for cellular DNA repair. It is thought that skin cells are therefore most vulnerable to UV radiation after prolonged periods of sun avoidance, when the melanin content and DNA-repair capacity are low. In addition, melanocytes are more resistant to

25

UV-induced apoptosis than keratinocytes and hence are more likely to survive highly damaging exposures and undergo mutations as a result. Perhaps, for these combined reasons, intermittent UV radiation is more important in the development of melanoma than of SCC. Unlike the melanocyte, the keratinocyte is unlikely to survive high-dose radiation; instead, recurrent low-dose UV radiation may gradually allow mutated clones to develop. Basal cells, the least differentiated of the epidermal keratinocytes, are likely to have a resistance to apoptosis intermediate to that of melanocytes and the suprabasilar keratinocytes from which SCC develop. This level of resistance would explain the epidemiological association of BCC with intermittent UV exposure as well as with chronic UV exposure.

Key points – pathogenesis

- Cells have many cancer-prevention mechanisms. Usually, several of them must be impaired in a single cell before uncontrolled (malignant) growth ensues.
- Cells lose anticancer defenses through mutation or decreased expression of the responsible gene products.
- Cancers usually contain a combination of mutations in proto-oncogenes (which create an oncogene and continuous positive-growth signaling) and in tumor suppressor genes (which disable the cellular 'brakes' or negative-growth signaling).
- Very rarely, mutations occur spontaneously. Far more often they result from exposure to DNA-damaging agents (carcinogens).
- Heritable disorders with a high risk of skin cancers are the result of mutations in the germline that either reduce DNA-repair capacity or compromise one of the important growth regulatory pathways in the cell.
- For skin, the major carcinogen is ultraviolet irradiation.

Key references

Gilchrest BA, Eller MS, Geller AC, Yaar M. The pathogenesis of melanoma induced by ultraviolet radiation. *N Engl J Med* 1999;340:1341–8.

Grossman D, Leffell DJ. The molecular basis of nonmelanoma skin cancer: new understanding. *Arch Dermatol* 1997;133:1263–70.

Tsao H. Genetics of nonmelanoma skin cancer. *Arch Dermatol* 2001;137:1486–92.

Clinical assessment is fundamental to the diagnostic process and begins with the patient history. A story of changing, enlarging and irritating lesions should alert suspicion. Patients who present with a skin cancer invariably describe a growth that is changing. It is reassuring to hear that a lesion is longstanding and is not changing.

Rigorous systematic clinical examination is mandatory to elicit key morphologic features (size, shape, symmetry, surface, margin, color, texture) of benign or malignant skin tumors. Primary care providers should consider early referral to a dermatologist for evaluation of any concerning lesion.

A clear diagnosis of a skin tumor is usually attained after clinical assessment, but histology is regarded as the gold standard.

The dermascope/dermatoscope, or surface microscope, is a handheld instrument that assists with the examination of cutaneous lesions. Generally, this light magnification system has a fixed magnification of ×10. Oil is usually applied to the skin lesion to reduce light refraction; however, newer systems with cross-polarized light enable examination without oil. The role of the dermascope is still evolving, but is of growing importance as the sensitivity and specificity of individual signs and patterns are described.

Biopsy and histology

Biopsy and histology are integral to the diagnosis of skin cancer.

Shave biopsy. When the skin lesion is pedunculated or only appears to involve the epidermis and upper dermis, a superficial slice of skin can be removed with a scalpel or razor blade. Sutures are not usually required and electrodesiccation or aluminum chloride may be applied to achieve hemostasis. The procedure leaves only a small scab that heals in 2–4 weeks.

Punch biopsy. Dermatologists are enthusiasts for this biopsy, and use it for suspected skin dermatoses and cancers. A circular blade attached to a handle is rotated through the skin, capturing a core of tissue from the epidermis to the subcutaneous fat. The core is removed and sent to the laboratory for histological assessment. Once the biopsy has been taken, the residual skin defect can be closed with sutures or adhesive strips. Alternatively, the wound can be left to heal on its own without stitches. A range of skin biopsy diameters is available, but in most situations a punch biopsy diameter of 3–6 mm is appropriate.

Excisional biopsy involves the removal of the entire lesion. The excision is usually elliptical. Excisional biopsy is the favored investigation for suspected melanomas in the UK, New Zealand and Australia. This technique allows the pathologist to evaluate the entire lesion.

Incisional biopsy involves removing an ellipse of tissue using a surgical blade, so that a proportion of the lesion can be sent for histological assessment. The remaining defect is usually repaired with sutures. This procedure is used when an excisional biopsy is technically challenging, such as in a large lentigo maligna melanoma.

Benign lesions
Acquired melanocytic nevi usually become apparent after the age of 12, and the numbers increase over the next 20 years before they start to dissipate. There are several types of acquired nevi:
- junctional
- compound
- intradermal
- halo
- pigmented spindle cell nevus of Reed
- Spitz
- blue.

Junctional nevi usually develop in adolescents, compound nevi in young adults and intradermal nevi in older adults. This observation has led to the hypothesis that throughout life the nevomelanocyte composition progresses from a junctional nevus to a compound nevus and then on to an intradermal nevus.

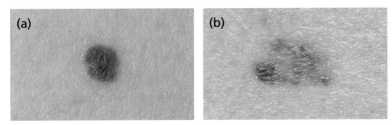

Figure 3.1 Junctional nevus: a flat, pigmented lesion, usually < 6 mm in diameter.

Junctional nevus most commonly arises in childhood and early adulthood. It is a flat sharply demarcated pigmented lesion, usually with a diameter of less than 6 mm (Figure 3.1). Junctional nevi often develop on palms and soles and tend to maintain the normal skin markings. Histologically, discrete nests of nevomelanocytes can be found in contact with the basal layer of the epidermis.

Compound nevus is a slightly elevated well-delineated pigmented lesion, most commonly found in adults (Figure 3.2). It tends to have a uniform color in the range of tan to dark brown. A proportion of the nevomelanocytes are free within the papillary dermis, whereas others are in contact with the overlying epidermal basal layer.

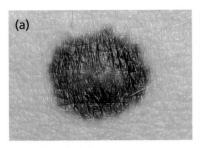

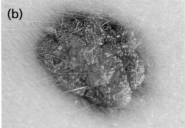

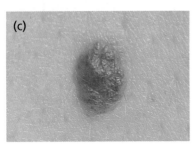

Figure 3.2 Compound nevus: an elevated well-delineated pigmented lesion, which tends to have a uniform color, ranging from tan to dark brown.

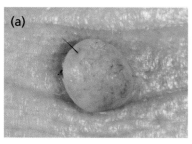

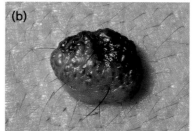

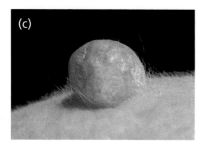

Figure 3.3 Intradermal nevus: a fleshy nodule or skin tag with minimal pigmentation, commonly found on the face.

Intradermal nevus tends to be a fleshy nodule or skin tag, with minimal pigmentation, commonly found on the face of older adults (Figure 3.3). Histological examination shows that the nevomelanocyte nests are free within the dermis and there is no involvement of the overlying epidermis.

Halo nevus, also termed Sutton's nevus, has a characteristic ring of hypopigmentation encircling the central pigmented nevus (Figure 3.4). The pigment loss is a consequence of an autoimmune assault on the compound nevus. This nevus, if not excised, will involute spontaneously over a few months; however, the depigmentation may

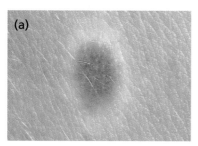

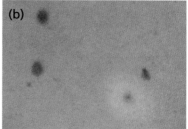

Figure 3.4 Halo nevus: (a) with a ring of hypopigmentation encircling the central pigmented nevus; (b) among multiple nevi on the back.

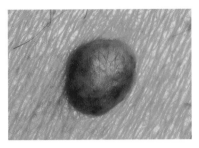

Figure 3.5 Spitz nevus: a rapidly growing, firm, orange-red papule, which commonly presents on the face.

persist for some years. Halo nevi most frequently develop on the trunks of adolescents and young adults.

Pigmented spindle cell nevus of Reed is a blue-black heavily pigmented nevus, seen more commonly in women than men, often on the thigh. Histologically, these lesions are comprised of spindle nevus cells with highly concentrated melanin.

Spitz nevus presents classically as a rapidly growing firm orange-red papule on the face. This compound nevus variant develops principally in children and young adults. It can be difficult to differentiate histologically from melanoma, and pathologists must exercise extreme caution if making the diagnosis in older individuals (Figure 3.5).

Blue nevus is a small uniform lesion of an intense black-blue color. It may be a macule, papule or plaque (Figure 3.6). Blue nevi are thought to arise from dermal melanocytes that did not complete their migration from the neural crest to the dermoepidermal junction during embryology.

(a)

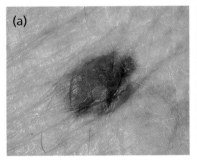

(b)

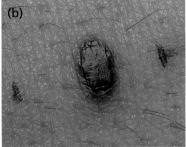

Figure 3.6 Blue nevus: a small, uniform lesion of an intense black-blue color, presenting as a macule, papule or plaque.

Seborrheic keratosis is a benign lesion generally seen in older individuals. It arises from epidermal keratinocytes and is variable in its clinical presentation (Figure 3.7). The lesion is usually elevated, warty and hyperkeratotic, and tends to reach a diameter of 10–30 mm.

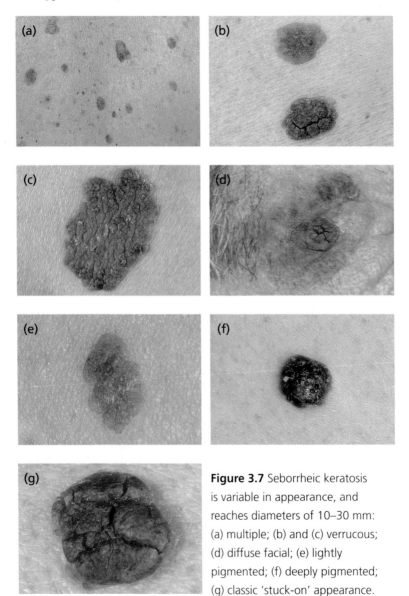

Figure 3.7 Seborrheic keratosis is variable in appearance, and reaches diameters of 10–30 mm: (a) multiple; (b) and (c) verrucous; (d) diffuse facial; (e) lightly pigmented; (f) deeply pigmented; (g) classic 'stuck-on' appearance.

Although generally uniform, the color may range from light brown to black. These are not melanocytic lesions: they obtain their pigment from melanosomes transferred to the keratinocytes from melanocytes. Seborrheic keratoses can be differentiated clinically from melanocytic lesions because they have a verrucous surface, contain keratin horns and have an elevated 'stuck-on' appearance.

Dermatofibroma. This benign dermal tumor presents as a firm papule or nodule, primarily on the limbs (Figure 3.8). The lesion has clear demarcation and ranges from a yellowish color to a dark purplish brown. The color is usually uniform, although there may be increased circumferential pigmentation.

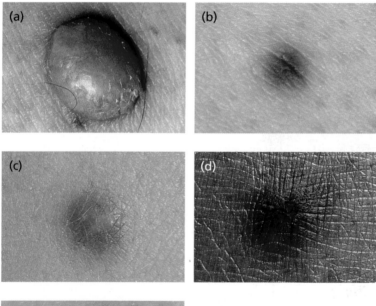

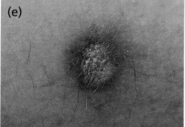

Figure 3.8 Dermatofibroma: a benign dermal tumor that presents as a firm papule or nodule, primarily on the limbs: (a) on ankle; (b) on abdomen; (c) well demarcated; (d) deeply pigmented; (e) with increased peripheral pigmentation.

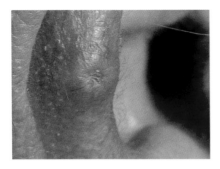

Figure 3.9 Chondrodermatitis nodularis helicis – a painful, benign nodule on the helix of the ear.

Chondrodermatitis nodularis helicis is a small benign but painful papule on the helix of the ear (Figure 3.9)

Premalignant lesions

Actinic (solar) keratosis is a benign scaly patch, papule or plaque that develops on sun-damaged skin. The lesions may be multiple, and arise predominantly on the face and dorsal aspects of the hands and forearms (Figure 3.10). An individual actinic keratosis characteristically fluctuates in size and can resolve spontaneously.

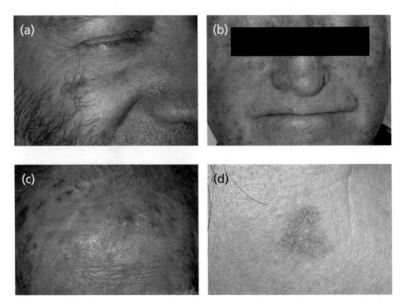

Figure 3.10 Actinic keratosis: a benign scaly patch, papule or plaque that develops on sun-damaged skin: (a) cheek; (b) face; (c) forehead; (d) temple.

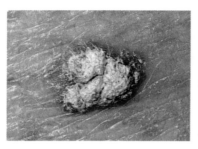

Figure 3.11 Bowenoid actinic keratosis – a small, irregular, keratotic lesion on sun-damaged skin; histology may be necessary to rule out a diagnosis of carcinoma in lesions that lack the characteristic features of an actinic keratosis.

Approximately 5% of lesions progress to squamous cell carcinoma (SCC) over time.

The diagnosis of an actinic keratosis is predominantly clinical. Histology of the lesion is appropriate when the clinical features are not characteristic, and it is important to exclude a cutaneous carcinoma (Figure 3.11). Actinic keratoses present in immunocompromised patients, such as organ-transplant recipients and those with HIV infection or chronic lymphocytic leukemia (Figure 3.12). A biopsy is also useful if the actinic keratosis has not responded to standard therapy. The lesions can be easily sampled using a punch biopsy or curette.

Histologically, there is focal parakeratosis, a slight thickening of the epidermis, loss of granular layer and variable alteration in the ordered epidermal architecture.

Keratoacanthoma is a distinctive tumor that presents as a rapidly growing self-resolving hyperkeratotic nodule (Figure 3.13). The lesion

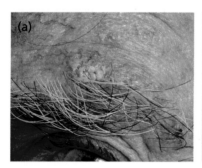
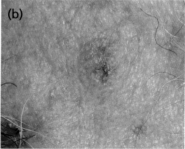

Figure 3.12 Florid actinic keratoses in a patient with chronic lymphocytic leukemia.

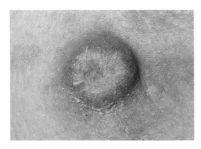

Figure 3.13 Keratoacanthoma on the cheek; this type of lesion is best regarded as a form of squamous cell carcinoma and should be treated as such.

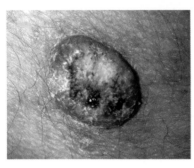

Figure 3.14 A keratoacanthoma-like squamous cell carcinoma.

usually develops on sun-exposed skin. Although some may be benign and involute spontaneously, it can be very difficult to differentiate keratoacanthoma from SCC, both clinically (Figure 3.14) and histologically. It is probably best regarded as a variant of squamous carcinoma. Keratoacanthoma is discussed in detail on pages 48–9.

Congenital melanocytic nevi (CMN) are a type of nevus present at birth. They can be divided into three subgroups depending on size:

- small CMN, with a widest projected adult diameter of less than 1.5 cm (Figure 3.15)
- medium CMN, with a projected adult size of between 1.5 and 20 cm (Figure 3.16)
- giant or large CMN, with a widest projected adult diameter of more than 20 cm.

In infancy, congenital nevi are generally a light-brown color; they may darken or lighten with age. These nevi tend to exhibit a mammillated surface and terminal hair follicles (Figure 3.17), and their borders are usually well demarcated. The larger CMN may have associated multiple nevi, also termed satellite nevi.

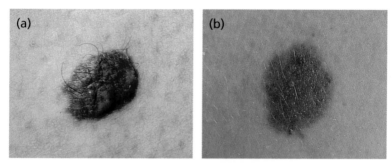

Figure 3.15 (a, b) Small congenital melanocytic nevi: widest diameter < 1.5 cm, with well-demarcated borders. Generally, light brown in infancy, darkening with age.

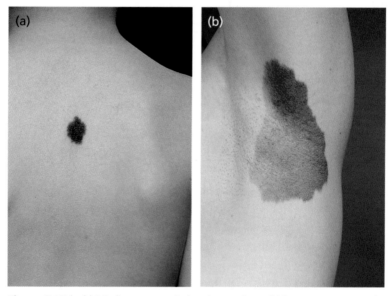

Figure 3.16 (a, b) Medium congenital melanocytic nevi (diameter 1.5–20 cm).

Congenital nevi have a greater risk of malignant transformation than acquired nevi. The highest risks are found with large or giant CMN, particularly those on the torso or where the projected adult size is greater than 40 cm in diameter. In this group the malignancy usually arises in the first 5–10 years of life and melanoma frequently develops within the nevus. However, it is not uncommon for patients to present with extracutaneous primary or metastatic disease.

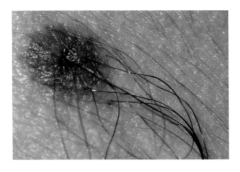

Figure 3.17 A small congenital nevus with a characteristic mammillated surface and terminal hair follicles.

Speckled lentiginous nevus (nevus spilus) may also be present at birth (Figure 3.18). Clinical examination reveals the characteristic hyperpigmented speckles within a light-brown macule, which distinguish this lesion from CMN.

Atypical nevus syndrome. Clinically, an atypical nevus can resemble a superficial spreading melanoma. Atypical nevi display varied pigmentation and irregular borders, and often have diameters of more than 10 mm (Figure 3.19). The nevi sometimes develop in unusual sites (Figure 3.20), and they often occur as multiple lesions (Figure 3.21), unlike melanomas, which usually present as single lesions. People with atypical nevi have an increased risk of developing melanoma.

Lentigo maligna (Hutchinson's freckle) is a benign pigmented lesion that begins as a small freckle and slowly enlarges. These brown patches have an irregular border and variegated coloration (Figure 3.22). They arise on sun-exposed skin, usually the head or neck, and develop mainly in people over 60 years old. They can grow

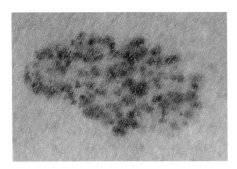

Figure 3.18 Speckled lentiginous nevus (nevus spilus) – characteristic hyperpigmented speckles within a light-brown macule.

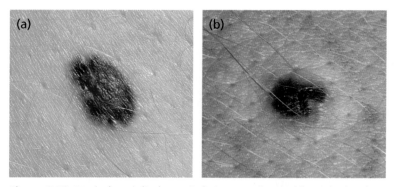

Figure 3.19 Atypical nevi display varied pigmentation and irregular borders.

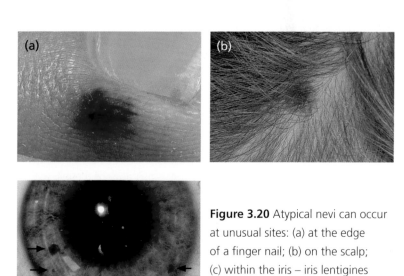

Figure 3.20 Atypical nevi can occur at unusual sites: (a) at the edge of a finger nail; (b) on the scalp; (c) within the iris – iris lentigines (arrowed).

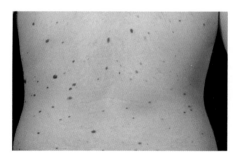

Figure 3.21 Atypical nevus syndrome, with characteristic multiple lesions.

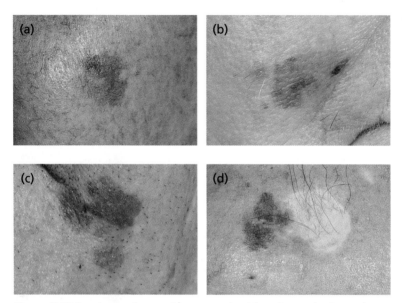

Figure 3.22 Lentigo maligna: a brown patch with variegated color and irregular borders: (a)–(c) on the face; (d) a recurrent lentigo maligna on the scalp.

and darken very slowly. Dark nodules or new indurated pigmented papules may arise after a variable period of time, a sign of malignant transformation. Approximately 5% of these lesions progress to lentigo maligna melanoma, a tumor with metastatic potential (see page 56; also, photographic documentation of progression at www.lentigomalignamelanoma.info).

A biopsy is essential to diagnose lentigo maligna, as the differential diagnosis includes benign pigmented patches such as solar and senile lentigines (Figure 3.23). As with all suspect pigmented lesions, these

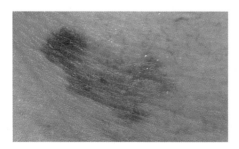

Figure 3.23 A senile lentigo, which has blander, more even, pigmentation than lentigo maligna.

41

are best sampled by an excisional biopsy with a narrow margin. If the lesion is too large for an excisional biopsy, an incisional biopsy may be appropriate. However, the portion of the tumor sampled with an incisional biopsy may not be representative of the entire lesion. The histology of lentigo maligna is discussed in the section on lentigo maligna melanoma (see page 56).

Malignant lesions

Basal cell carcinoma (BCC) is the most common human malignancy; it accounts for approximately three-quarters of all skin cancers. The majority of BCCs arise on the head and neck (Figure 3.24).

BCC can be subdivided into a number of clinicopathological variants:

- nodular (solid)
- micronodular
- superficial
- pigmented
- adenocystic
- morpheic (sclerosing)
- infiltrative
- basosquamous.

Solid or nodular basal cell carcinoma is the most common variant, and develops predominantly on the face (Figure 3.25). A solid BCC initially appears as a translucent pearly nodule that slowly enlarges. Classically, the lesion is shiny and well defined, containing dilated superficial capillaries (Figure 3.26). These vessels are located in the

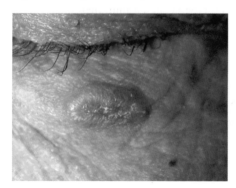

Figure 3.24 Basal cell carcinoma usually arises on the head and neck.

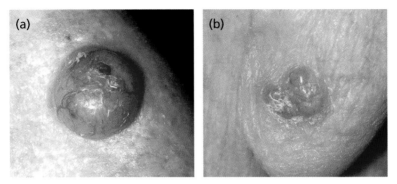

Figure 3.25 Nodular basal cell carcinoma: (a) on the nose, displaying superficial capillaries; (b) on the earlobe.

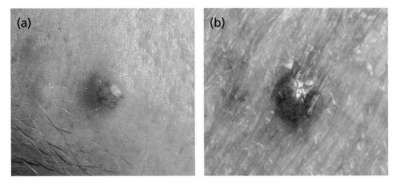

Figure 3.26 Nodular or solid basal cell carcinoma presents as a shiny well-defined papule or nodule containing dilated superficial capillaries.

thin layer of epithelium that covers the tumor, an area that may periodically scale, erode or crust.

When the diameter of a BCC is greater than 5 mm, there is a tendency for central ulceration to occur. A large nodular BCC often has a characteristic pearly rolled appearance at the lesion periphery (Figure 3.27), which can be accentuated by stretching the skin.

Micronodular basal cell carcinoma resembles solid BCC but differs histologically and has a higher risk of recurrence after treatment.

Superficial basal cell carcinoma, which usually arises on the trunk, accounts for 10% of all BCCs (Figure 3.28). The lesions extend superficially and are well defined with a thread-like raised edge. The thin plaques may display central atrophy or scaling, making it difficult

43

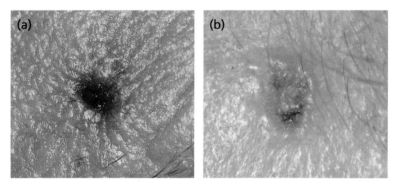

Figure 3.27 Ulcerated basal cell carcinoma: (a) ulceration may occur when the nodule diameter reaches more than 5 mm; (b) large nodule exhibiting a classic rolled pearly edge.

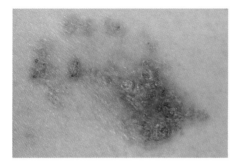

Figure 3.28 A superficial basal cell carcinoma on the back, exhibiting a thread-like raised edge; the thin plaques may display central atrophy or scaling.

to differentiate them from in situ SCCs. Peripheral islands of tumor and pigmentation are not uncommon.

Pigmented basal cell carcinoma is usually a superficial, micronodular or nodular variant that demonstrates obvious pigmentation (Figure 3.29). It may be brown, red or black, and either completely or irregularly pigmented. The pigmentation is a result of trapped melanin or altered blood composition, and occurs in 2–5% of all BCCs.

Adenocystic basal cell carcinoma tends to present clinically as a diffuse plaque with a rolled edge. Cystic components of this tumor have a more translucent appearance.

Morpheic basal cell carcinoma is rare, accounting for only 2% of all BCCs. Occurring almost exclusively on the face, the lesions can be difficult to identify. Morpheic BCC presents as an indurated scar-like

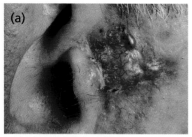

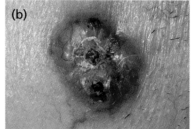

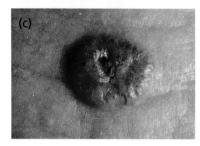

Figure 3.29 Pigmented nodular basal cell carcinoma (BCC); the BCC in (c) is ulcerated.

plaque with waxy yellow coloration (Figure 3.30). The margins are ill-defined, and on palpation the BCC is usually considerably larger than it appears on visual inspection (Figure 3.31).

Infiltrative basal cell carcinoma is clinically similar to the morpheic variant in that they both have indistinct borders. However, histologically, infiltrative tumor cells are not embedded in the dense fibrous stroma, as occurs in morpheic BCC. Both of these BCC variants are difficult to treat and have higher recurrence rates.

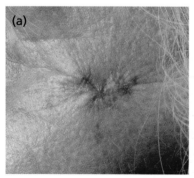

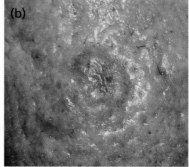

Figure 3.30 Morpheic basal cell carcinoma: (a) displaying scar-like features; (b) presenting as an indurated plaque.

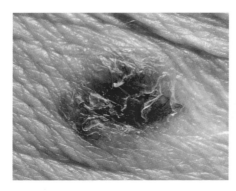

Figure 3.31 A combined solid and morpheic basal cell carcinoma.

Basosquamous basal cell carcinoma is described as having histological features of both BCC and SCC. Some pathologists use this term when it is difficult to distinguish between keratinizing BCC and poorly differentiated SCC. Clinically, the lesions resemble SCC more than BCC and there is controversy over whether these lesions are actually SCC rather than BCC variants.

Sebaceous nevus complicated by basal cell carcinoma tends to present initially as a nodule within the papillomatous nevus. The risk of developing an associated BCC increases with age, although it has been reported in teenagers.

Nevoid basal cell carcinoma syndrome (Gorlin's syndrome). Patients with Gorlin's syndrome have a mutation – inherited or arising spontaneously in early embryologic development – in one copy of the patched 1 gene (*PTCH1*). When the remaining normal copy of the gene is damaged (e.g. by ultraviolet [UV] or X-ray exposure) a cancer develops.

Classically, patients have multiple BCCs, which are located most commonly on the eyelids, nose, cheeks and forehead, often at symmetric sites (Figure 3.32). Although these tumors may be present at birth or develop in infancy, they are not usually identified until adolescence.

The BCCs are predominantly nodular and have a benign course, similar to sporadic BCC. Other clinical features of Gorlin's syndrome include palmoplantar hyperkeratosis and depressions in the skin surface (pits) (Figure 3.33), dental cysts, frontal bossing and abnormalities of the vertebrae and ribs. These associations reflect the

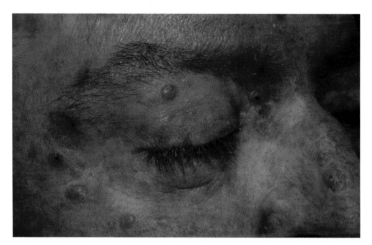

Figure 3.32 Multiple basal cell carcinomas located on the eyelids and cheeks of a patient with Gorlin's syndrome.

important role of the *PTCH1* gene in skeletal development as well as in skin maintenance.

Diagnosis. Clinical assessment is often sufficient to make the diagnosis, so treatment can be initiated straight away. However, there are situations in which it is difficult to differentiate a BCC clinically from other lesions such as sebaceous hyperplasia (Figure 3.34), dermatofibroma (see Figure 3.8), SCC and amelanotic melanoma (see Figure 3.50). A biopsy is helpful when there is clinical doubt and before referral for specialist treatment.

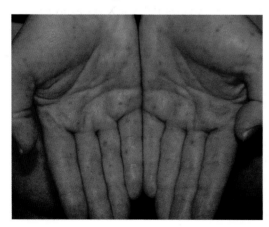

Figure 3.33
Palmoplantar hyperkeratosis and pits in a patient with Gorlin's syndrome.

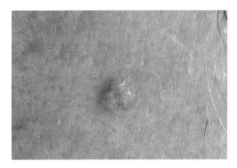

Figure 3.34 Sebaceous hyperplasia – a benign condition in which single or multiple small yellowish papules develop, usually on the face.

Treatments such as radiotherapy, Mohs surgery, photodynamic therapy and topical therapies generally require a baseline histological diagnosis. A biopsy also provides information on the BCC subtype, which may direct management and assist with prognosis.

Histology. The histological features of a BCC vary with the different subtypes. BCC is composed of islands, or nests, of basaloid cells in the dermis, and there is often some attachment to the undersurface of the epidermis (Figure 3.35). The tumor cells have hyperchromatic nuclei with multiple mitoses and sparse cytoplasm. The neoplastic cells in superficial BCC are attached to the epidermis, and are confined to the papillary dermis. In morpheic BCC, the narrow strands of tumor cells are embedded in a dense fibrous stroma.

Metastasis. Most lesions of BCC are small. However, if the presentation is delayed, these tumors can extend from the skin into soft tissue, cartilage and bone. BCC has been known to metastasize on very rare occasions. The most common sites of metastasis are lymph nodes, lung and brain.

Keratoacanthoma is a distinctive tumor that presents as a rapidly growing self-resolving hyperkeratotic nodule (see Figure 3.13). The lesions usually develop on sun-exposed skin and have three clinical stages:
- proliferation – an initial stage of 2–4 weeks in which the lesion enlarges to more than 20 mm in diameter
- maturation for a few months
- involution – final tumor reabsorption over a further 4–6 months and expulsion of the keratin-filled core.

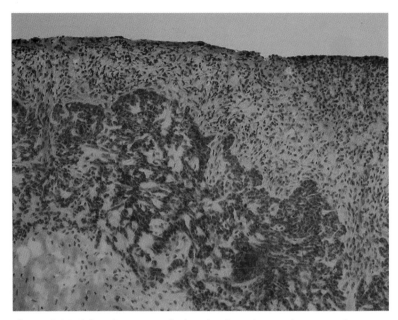

Figure 3.35 Light microscopy of a basal cell carcinoma demonstrating nests of basaloid cells within the dermis.

Clinically, a keratoacanthoma begins as a smooth papule with slightly erythematous surrounding skin. During the maturation stage, it develops a dome shape with a central keratin plug (Figure 3.36). This plug is later expelled. An atrophic scar often persists after resolution.

Although keratoacanthoma may be a benign tumor, it can be very difficult to differentiate from SCC, both clinically (see Figure 3.14) and histologically. The potential of keratoacanthoma to develop into SCC in the immunosuppressed population is well known. There have also been reports of this phenomenon in non-immunosuppressed individuals. Keratoacanthoma is perhaps best regarded as a variant of SCC.

Keratoacanthomas are usually removed by surgical excision. Histological examination of a keratoacanthoma reveals a crater lined with well-differentiated squamous epithelium containing a large central keratin plug. The central keratin component enlarges as the keratoacanthoma matures.

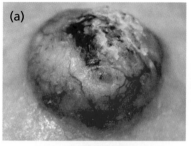

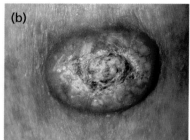

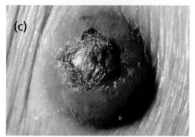

Figure 3.36 Keratoacanthoma has a characteristic central keratin plug.

Squamous cell carcinoma develops on photodamaged skin, usually at sites with the highest exposure to UV radiation. These include the face, neck and dorsum of the hands and forearms. In men, commonly affected sites are the lower lip and pinna, whereas in women the lower legs are frequently involved. SCC can also develop within chronic ulcers or in other situations where cells are constantly stimulated to divide. Genital SCC is strongly associated with pre-existing SCC or 'high risk' human papillomavirus (HPV) types.

In situ (intraepidermal). Here, the abnormal keratinocytes are confined to the epidermis. Bowen's disease, first described in 1912, is the most common form of in situ SCC. Classic Bowen's disease presents as a persistent slightly scaly well-demarcated erythematous plaque (Figure 3.37).

The lesions are often isolated and slow growing. Approximately 3% of intraepidermal SCC progress to invasive SCC (Figure 3.38).

Other forms of in situ SCC include those associated with local HPV infection, such as bowenoid papulosis and erythroplasia of Queyrat (Figure 3.39). In bowenoid papulosis, men and women develop polymorphic velvety warty papules and plaques in the anogenital region. Erythroplasia of Queyrat is a form of penile intraepithelial

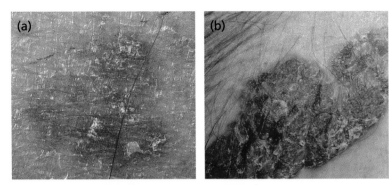

Figure 3.37 Bowen's disease presents as a persistent slightly scaly well-demarcated erythematous plaque: (a) on the calf; (b) on the inner thigh.

neoplasia of the uncircumcised male, in which red shiny patches or plaques form on the glans penis and prepuce.

The diagnosis of in situ SCC is often made clinically. However, a biopsy is helpful in confirming the diagnosis, particularly as many treatments are non-surgical. Tissue sampling with a punch biopsy is adequate and appropriate where there is suspicion of invasive malignancy.

The histology of in situ SCC is of atypical keratinocytes throughout the full thickness of the epidermis. The maturation of the epidermis is

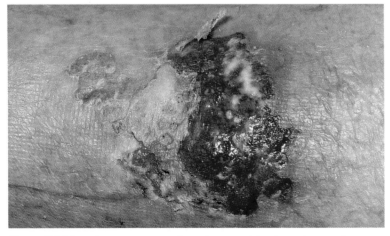

Figure 3.38 Invasive squamous cell carcinoma arising in a plaque of Bowen's disease.

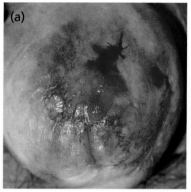

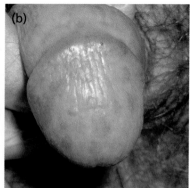

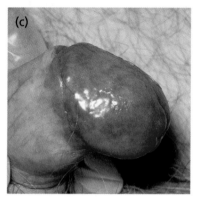

Figure 3.39 (a) Bowen's disease and squamous cell carcinoma (SCC) of the glans penis. A punch biopsy showed high-grade dysplasia, and a deep elliptical biopsy revealed invasive SCC; (b) bowenoid papulosis of the glans penis in a patient with HIV; (c) erythroplasia of Queyrat – SCC in situ of the glans penis.

disorderly, and there is usually overlying parakeratosis and hyperkeratosis.

Invasive squamous cell carcinoma often arises in an area of pre-existing actinic keratosis. The first suspect sign is an ill-defined firm indurated lesion (Figure 3.40). This is usually nodular, but it may be plaque-like, verrucous or ulcerated. The tumor is often a yellow-red color with a crusted cap, and will continue to enlarge (Figure 3.41). The surrounding tissue is often inflamed. When mucosal sites are affected, individuals present with non-healing erosions, ulcers or fissures that may bleed intermittently.

Verrucous carcinoma (Buschke–Löwenstein tumor) is a rare low-grade well-differentiated SCC. These tumors are warty, vegetating and slow growing. They are typically found in the anogenital region or on the plantar aspect of the foot, although they may also develop in

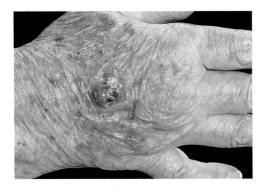

Figure 3.40 Invasive squamous cell carcinoma arising in an area of actinic damage on the dorsum of the hand.

the oral cavity. They rarely metastasize. Other precursors for invasive SCC include:

- actinic keratosis
- in situ SCC
- cutaneous horns
- chronic inflammation or scars.

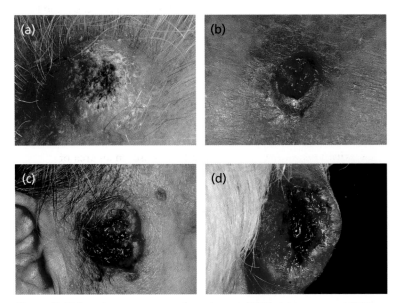

Figure 3.41 Invasive squamous cell carcinoma (SCC): (a) a recurrent SCC on the forehead; (b) an ulcerated SCC with surrounding inflammation; (c) a large crusted and ulcerated SCC on the temple; (d) a poorly differentiated SCC on the ear.

53

Invasive SCC can develop in chronic scars, sinuses or ulcers, including, for example, in erythema ab igne (a red-brown hyperpigmentation of the skin caused by chronic local exposure to heat), hidradenitis suppurativa and venous ulceration (Marjolin's ulcer).

Tumors arising in scars or areas of chronic inflammation have an increased risk of metastasizing. There is also an elevated metastatic risk in SCC developing on the lip, ear and non-sun-exposed sites.

In invasive SCC, the diagnosis is suspected clinically and established histologically. A punch, incisional or, preferably, an excisional biopsy can be used.

Histological examination of an invasive SCC reveals dermal nests of squamous epithelial cells arising from the epidermis (Figure 3.42). There may be associated formations of keratin. The atypical squamous cells have large nuclei with abundant eosinophilic cytoplasm.

The histology report should include the histopathological pattern or subtype of SCC, the degree of differentiation, the level of dermal invasion and the presence of perineural, vascular or lymphatic invasion. Information on the margins of the excised tumor is also necessary.

Staging. The American Joint Committee on Cancer (AJCC) recently published a new staging system for cutaneous SCC, which incorporates tumor-specific (T) staging features (Table 3.1).

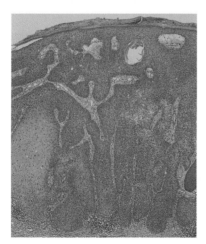

Figure 3.42 Light microscopy of a moderately differentiated invasive squamous cell carcinoma in which dermal nests of atypical squamous epithelial cells arise from the epidermis.

TABLE 3.1

American Joint Committee on Cancer cutaneous squamous cell carcinoma staging system

Stage	T	N	M
0	In situ	N0	M0
I	T1	N0	M0
II	T2	N0	M0
III	T3	N0 or N1	M0
	T1 or T2	N1	M0
IV	T1, 2 or 3	N2	M0
	Any T	N3	M0
	T4	Any N	M0
	Any T	Any N	M1

Key:

T0 – No evidence of primary tumor.

T1 – Tumor ≤ 2 cm in greatest dimension with fewer than two high-risk features.

T2 – Tumor > 2 cm in greatest dimension with/without one additional high-risk feature or any size with ≥ 2 high-risk features.

T3 –Tumor with invasion of maxilla, mandible, orbit, or temporal bone.

T4 –Tumor with invasion of skeleton (axial or appendicular) or perineural invasion of skull base.

N0 – No regional lymph node metastasis.

N1 – Metastasis in single ipsilateral lymph node, ≤ 3 cm in greatest dimension.

N2 – Metastasis in single ipsilateral lymph node, > 3 cm but not > 6 cm in greatest dimension; or in mutiple ipsilateral lymph nodes, none > 6 cm in greatest dimension; or in bilateral or contralateral lymph nodes, none > 6 cm in greatest dimension.

N2a – Metastasis in single ipsilateral lymph node, > 3 cm but not > 6 cm in greatest dimension.

N2b – Metastasis in multiple ipsilateral lymph nodes, none > 6 cm in greatest dimension.

N2c – Metastasis in bilateral or contralateral lymph nodes, none > 6 cm in greatest dimension.

N3 – Metastasis in lymph node, > 6 cm.

M0 – No distant metastasis.

M1 – Present distant metastasis.

Adapted from Farasat S et al. 2011

Melanoma subtypes have distinct clinical presentations; the incidence of these subtypes is shown in Figure 3.43. However, the history of an enlarging and changing pigmented lesion is characteristic of most melanomas. Sun exposure is implicated in at least two-thirds of these malignancies.

Lentigo maligna melanoma is found predominantly on sun-exposed areas in older individuals. Around 90% of lesions occur on the head or neck. They develop from the preinvasive lentigo maligna (Hutchinson's melanotic freckle) (see pages 39 and 41–2; also, photographic documentation of progression at www.lentigomalignamelanoma.info).

After a variable period of time, the invasive phase develops within the lentigo maligna; when the neoplastic melanocytes have extended to the dermis it transforms into a lentigo maligna melanoma (Figure 3.44). At this stage, the neoplasm has metastatic potential. Lentigo maligna melanoma can often be detected clinically as a densely pigmented nodule within the original macular lesion. These nodules can grow rapidly.

Superficial spreading melanoma accounts for approximately 80% of all melanoma. It is observed most frequently on the calves of women and the backs of men.

A typical superficial spreading melanoma is asymmetrical and irregularly outlined. It can be crusted, and presents in different shades of brown, black, red, blue or white (Figure 3.45). The tumor can expand both radially through the epidermis and vertically into the dermis over a period of months or years.

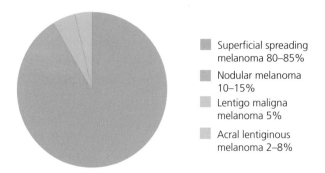

Superficial spreading melanoma 80–85%

Nodular melanoma 10–15%

Lentigo maligna melanoma 5%

Acral lentiginous melanoma 2–8%

Figure 3.43 Relative incidence of the melanoma subtypes.

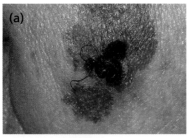

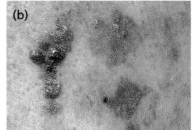

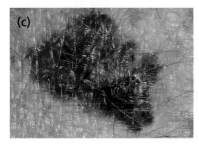

Figure 3.44 Lentigo maligna melanoma: (a) with surrounding lentigo maligna; (b) on a sun-exposed area; (c) complicating the inferior aspect of the lentigo maligna.

Nodular melanoma most frequently arises on the trunk and is first observed as a raised black or blue nodular growth (Figure 3.46). Such growths expand rapidly, and the overlying epidermis may ulcerate; it can be difficult to differentiate nodular melanomas from vascular tumors (Figure 3.47).

Acral lentiginous melanoma predominantly occurs in black populations and in people from South East Asia and the Indian subcontinent. Plantar melanoma is more common on the soles than on the palms. It begins as a macule that enlarges and develops a black elevated nodular component. Subungual malignant melanoma, with black pigmentation beneath the nail plate, is another form of acral lentiginous melanoma (Figure 3.48). The differential diagnosis includes hemorrhage (Figure 3.49) and fungal infection. Pigmentation of the nail fold ('Hutchinson's sign') is highly suggestive of melanoma.

Amelanotic melanoma is difficult to identify and should be included in the differential diagnosis of any rapidly growing nodule. Although the name suggests an absence of pigment, amelanotic melanoma usually does have some brown pigmentation to alert the physician to the correct diagnosis (Figure 3.50). These melanomas tend to display telangiectasia, and are usually more vascular than intradermal nevi.

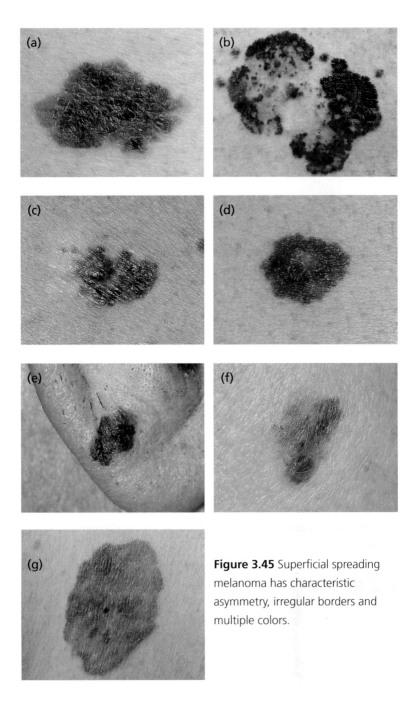

Figure 3.45 Superficial spreading melanoma has characteristic asymmetry, irregular borders and multiple colors.

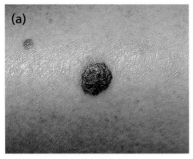

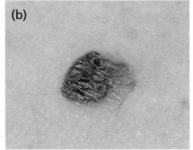

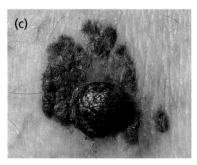

Figure 3.46 Nodular melanoma: (a) with characteristic blue-black pigmentation; (b) developed within a dysplastic nevus, with Breslow thickness 1.2 mm; (c) a combined nodular and superficial spreading melanoma.

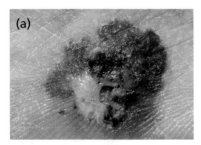

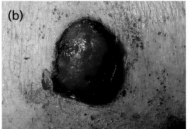

Figure 3.47 Nodular melanoma: (a) displaying crusting and ulceration; (b) with an amelanotic component – may be difficult to differentiate from a vascular tumor.

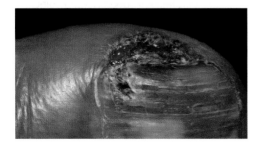

Figure 3.48 A subungual malignant melanoma exhibiting black pigmentation beneath the nail.

Figure 3.49 A subungual hematoma arising secondary to trauma – not to be confused with a subungual malignant melanoma (see Figure 3.48).

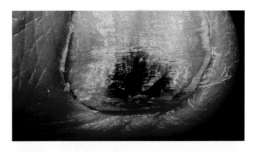

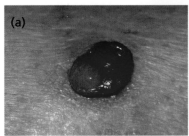
(a)

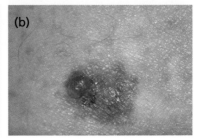
(b)

Figure 3.50 Amelanotic melanoma: (b) shows an amelanotic melanoma with a pigmented component, which can aid diagnosis.

Diagnosis. Early diagnosis of melanoma is essential, as the survival rate decreases with increasing tumor thickness. Clinical diagnosis of malignant melanoma can be difficult, as the differential diagnosis is wide, and includes nevi (see pages 29–32), seborrheic keratosis (see Figure 3.7), dermatofibroma (see Figure 3.8), pyogenic granuloma (Figure 3.51), vascular lesions and cutaneous metastases (Figure 3.52). The ABCDEF rule (Table 3.2) is a simple guide that can assist with identifying early melanomas. However, it is only a guide, and it should not be applied strictly – for example, early melanoma may be smaller than 6 mm and there may be no pigment in an amelanotic melanoma.

The Australia and New Zealand guidelines for managing melanoma promote the use of the seven-point checklist to assist with clinical diagnosis (Table 3.3). This system emphasizes the importance of irregular color or shape and change in size in the identification of suspect lesions.

Dermoscopy. The dermascope can assist with the clinical diagnosis of melanoma, enabling examination of the anatomic structures of the epidermis, dermoepidermal junction and superficial papillary dermis.

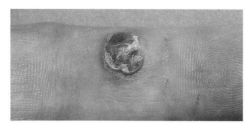

Figure 3.51 Pyogenic granuloma.

Figure 3.52 Cutaneous metastases arising from an internal malignancy.

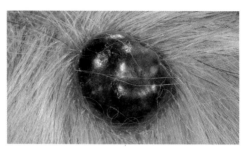

Several pigment patterns that can be seen with this instrument are suggestive of melanoma. The dermascopic findings can be put into an algorithm to calculate the likelihood of a malignant melanoma. Examples of algorithms include the ABCD rule of dermoscopy, the seven-point checklist and Menzies' scoring method (Table 3.4). These have been developed from the initial technique of pattern analysis, and all are recognized as valid methods for evaluating pigmented lesions with dermoscopy. A meta-analysis comparing dermoscopy with naked-eye examination for the diagnosis of melanoma concluded that, for experienced operators, dermoscopy gave a more accurate

TABLE 3.2

Clinical features of melanoma – the ABCDEF rule

A	Lesion asymmetry
B	Irregular border
C	Multiple colors
D	Diameter > 6 mm
E	Evolution/elevation
F	'Funny' mole

TABLE 3.3

Seven-point checklist for melanoma

Melanoma should be suspected if there is any one major feature or any combination of three minor features

Major features	Minor features
Change in size	Diameter > 6 mm
Irregular shape	Inflammation
Irregular color	Oozing
	Change in sensation

diagnosis. Although dermoscopy can improve diagnostic accuracy for the trained clinician, it has not yet been shown to increase the sensitivity of excision biopsy in malignant melanoma. Sequential digital dermoscopy imaging is a further tool available for monitoring pigmented lesions and recording change.

Biopsy. If there is suspicion of melanoma, a full-thickness excisional biopsy of the tumor should be performed. The UK, US and Australian and New Zealand melanoma guidelines recommend that the pigmented lesion under investigation should be excised initially with a narrow margin (1–3 mm) to the depth of subcutaneous fat. Punch and shave biopsies should not be used, as they interfere with histological staging. An incisional biopsy is occasionally appropriate in large lesions on the face suggestive of lentigo maligna or when sampling for subungual melanoma. Incisional biopsy has not been shown to have an adverse effect on survival. If there is suspicion of subungual melanoma then sufficient nail should be removed for the concerning lesion or nail matrix to be adequately biopsied.

Histopathological assessment is fundamental to the diagnosis of melanoma and should be performed by a pathologist who is experienced in diagnosing pigmented lesions. The histology also provides information on prognosis and directs the therapeutic intervention. The most important prognostic factor is the Breslow

thickness of a tumor; it is measured histologically from the top of the

TABLE 3.4

Menzies' scoring method for the dermascopic diagnosis of invasive melanoma

Melanoma is suspected in a lesion that does not have both reassuring features and has one or more 'worrying' feature

Reassuring features (absent in all melanomas)*

- **Symmetry of pattern** through the lesion's radial and longitudinal axes
- **Presence of a single color** – black, gray, blue, dark brown, tan and red are scored, but white is not scored as a color

Worrying features (specificity of > 85% for invasive melanoma)*

- **Blue-white veil** – an irregular, structureless area of confluent blue pigmentation with an overlying white 'ground-glass' haze
- **Multiple brown dots** – focal areas of well-defined dark-brown dots (not globules)
- **Pseudopods** – bulbous and often kinked projections found at the edge of a lesion directly connected to either the tumor body or pigmented network
- **Radial streaming** – asymmetrically arranged finger-like extensions at the edge of the lesion
- **Scar-like depigmentation** – areas of white, discrete, irregular extensions, not to be confused with hypo- or depigmentation caused by simple loss of melanin
- **Peripheral black dots/globules** – found at or near the edge of the lesion
- **Multiple (5–6) colors** – black, gray, blue, dark brown, tan and red are scored, but white is not scored as a color
- **Multiple blue/gray dots** – a 'pepper-like' pattern of blue or gray dots (not globules)
- **Broadened network** – pigmented network with irregular, thick 'cords', often seem focally thicker

*In Menzies' original training set (Menzies S et al. *Melanoma Res* 1996;6: 55–62).
Adapted from Menzies et al. *Arch Dermatol* 1996;132:1178–82.

granular layer to the deepest tumor cell. Information that should appear in the histopathology report is shown in Table 3.5.

The histopathological features of melanoma differ between subtypes. However, in general, the radial growth phase – the process by which a pigmented lesion extends horizontally – correlates with the proliferation of atypical melanocytes within the epidermis or papillary dermis. This is followed by the vertical growth phase, except in nodular melanoma, in which there is no radial growth phase.

In lentigo maligna, the atypical melanocytes are usually confined to the basal layer of the epidermis, where they occur singly or in nests, and may extend to the adnexal epithelium. This transforms to lentigo maligna melanoma when it develops an invasive component.

Superficial spreading melanoma is characterized by proliferating atypical melanocytes present at all levels of the epidermis.

Nodular melanoma is comprised of a dermal mass of melanoma cells and, although there may be some invasion to the overlying epidermis, the tumor does not have an intraepithelial component.

Physical examination. An individual recently diagnosed with melanoma requires a thorough physical examination to search for any lymphadenopathy, hepatomegaly or other suspect pigmented lesions. If any such abnormalities are identified on physical examination, further investigation is required. There is strong evidence that routine imaging

TABLE 3.5

Information that should be included in the melanoma histopathology report

• Tumor site	• Degree of tumor regression
• Surgical procedure undertaken	• Mitotic index
• Macroscopic examination and dimensions	• Presence of microsatellites
• Breslow thickness	• Statement on completeness of excision with margins
• Evidence of ulceration	• Tumor-infiltrating lymphocytes
• Degree of radial and/or vertical growth	• Lymphatic or vascular invasion
	• Perineural invasion
• Melanoma subtype	• Pathological staging

and blood tests have little, if any, value for the asymptomatic patient who has a normal physical examination and a Breslow thickness of 4 mm or less.

Staging. The AJCC provides a melanoma staging system that is widely accepted around the world. The British melanoma guidelines suggest that no further investigations are required for asymptomatic patients with stage I, II or IIIA disease. However, for those with stage IIIB or IIIC melanoma, CT scanning of the head, chest, abdomen and pelvis is recommended. This would normally exclude metastases, which is important in the pretreatment workup for lymph node dissection or regional chemotherapy. Furthermore, the guidelines recommend measurement of lactate dehydrogenase level for all patients with suspected stage IV disease, with consideration of entire body imaging for this group (Table 3.6).

Some clinicians are now using whole-body fluorine-18 fluorodeoxyglucose positron emission tomography (PET)/CT imaging for identifying melanoma metastases. This appears to have superior results when compared with conventional imaging. However, its exact role in melanoma management is yet to be determined.

Key points – clinical features and diagnosis

- Although there are a number of basal cell carcinoma (BCC) variants, the classic presentation is a pearly nodule (containing superficial dilated capillaries) that slowly enlarges and develops central ulceration.
- BCC can often be diagnosed on clinical examination alone; a biopsy is useful when there is uncertainty over the diagnosis, or before the patient is referred for specialist treatment.
- Invasive SCC usually arises in an area of pre-existing actinic keratosis and is an ill-defined firm yellow-red lesion. A biopsy is required to confirm the diagnosis.
- Melanoma presents as a new or pre-existing enlarging and changing pigmented lesion. Early diagnosis is imperative and is made by excisional biopsy.

TABLE 3.6

Cancer staging for cutaneous melanoma

Stage	Primary tumor (T)	Lymph nodes (N)	Metastases (M)
IA	≤ 1 mm, no ulceration, mitoses < 1/mm^2	–	–
IB	≤ 1 mm, with ulceration or mitoses ≥ 1/mm^2* 1.01–2 mm, no ulceration	–	–
IIA	1·01–2 mm, with ulceration 2·01–4 mm, no ulceration	–	–
IIB	2·01–4 mm, with ulceration > 4 mm, no ulceration	–	–
IIC	> 4 mm, with ulceration	–	–
IIIA	Any Breslow thickness, no ulceration	Micrometastases 1–3 nodes	–
IIIB	Any Breslow thickness, with ulceration	Micrometastases 1–3 nodes	–
	Any Breslow thickness, no ulceration	1–3 palpable metastatic nodes	
	Any Breslow thickness, no ulceration	No nodes, but in-transit or satellite metastasis/es	

CONTINUED

TABLE 3.6 CONTINUED

Stage	Primary tumor (T)	Lymph nodes (N)	Metastases (M)
IIIC	Any Breslow thickness, with ulceration	Up to 3 palpable lymph nodes	–
	Any Breslow thickness, with or without ulceration	≥ 4 nodes or matted nodes or in-transit disease + lymph nodes	
	Any Breslow thickness, with ulceration	No nodes, but in-transit or satellite metastasis/es	
IV, M1a	–	–	Skin, subcutaneous or distant nodal disease
IV, M1b	–	–	Lung metastases
IV, M1c	–	–	All other sites or any other sites of metastases with raised LDH

*In the rare circumstances where mitotic count cannot be accurately determined, a Clark level of invasion of either IV or V can be used to define TIB melanoma.
LDH, lactate dehydrogenase.
Adapted from Marsden JR et al. 2010 and Balch CM et al. 2009.

Key references

Bafounta M, Beauchet A, Aegerter P, Saiag P. Is dermoscopy (epiluminescence microscopy) useful for the diagnosis of melanoma? Results of a meta-analysis using techniques adapted to the evaluation of diagnostic tests. *Arch Dermatol* 2001;137:1343–50.

Balch CM, Gershenwald JE, Soong SJ et al. Final version of 2009 AJCC melanoma staging and classification. *J Clin Oncol* 2009;27:6199–206.

Bunker CB. Scientific evidence and expert clinical opinion for the investigation and management of stage I malignant melanoma. In: MacKie RM, Murray D, Rosin RD et al., eds. *The Effective Management of Malignant Melanoma.* London: Aesculapius Medical Press, 2001:37–44.

Farasat S, Yu SS, Neel VA et al. A new American Joint Committee on Cancer staging system for cutaneous squamous cell carcinoma: creation and rationale for inclusion of tumor (T) characteristics. *J Am Acad Dermatol* 2011;64:1051–9.

Heaphy MR Jr, Ackerman AB. The nature of solar keratosis: a critical review in historical perspective. *J Am Acad Dermatol* 2000;43:138–50.

Johr RH. Dermoscopy: alternative melanocytic algorithms – the ABCD rule of dermatoscopy, Menzies scoring method, and 7-point checklist. *Clin Dermatol* 2002;20:240–7.

Marsden JR, Newton-Bishop JA, Burrows L et al. Revised U.K. guidelines for the management of cutaneous melanoma 2010. *Br J Dermatol* 2010;163:238–56.

Menzies SW, Crotty KA, Ingvar C, McCarthy WH. *An Atlas of Surface Microscopy of Pigmented Skin Lesions: Dermoscopy*, 2nd edn. Sydney: McGraw-Hill, 2003.

Tsao H. Update on familial cancer syndromes and the skin. *J Am Acad Dermatol* 2000;42:939–69.

Vestergaard ME, Macaskill P, Holt PE, Menzies SW. Dermoscopy compared with naked-eye examination for the diagnosis of primary melanoma: a meta-analysis of studies performed in a clinical setting. *Br J Dermatol* 2008;159:669–76.

4 Management

Treatments

Most tumors are surgically excised. However, there are a number of different treatments that may be suitable for patients with premalignant or malignant cutaneous lesions. These include:
- topical preparations
- cryotherapy
- curettage and electrosurgery
- Mohs micrographic surgery
- photodynamic therapy (PDT) and lasers
- radiotherapy.

Topical therapies may be sufficient to treat premalignant and superficial malignant cutaneous lesions. They are discussed under management of actinic keratoses (pages 80–1).

Cryotherapy is an easily administered treatment for a number of cutaneous premalignant and malignant lesions. Of the cryogens, liquid nitrogen (which boils at −196°C) is the most effective for treating skin cancer; when it is used clinically, intra- and extracellular ice crystals form, causing cell rupture and tissue destruction. The liquid nitrogen, contained in a handheld unit, is applied to the skin via a spray or probe. It is best directed at areas with a diameter of 6 mm or less – small lesions or discrete areas within larger lesions. In this way, the epidermis and dermis are frozen effectively.

Some cryosurgeons prefer a continuous-freeze technique, whereas others apply the spray in pulses. The period in seconds during which the liquid nitrogen is applied and the number of freeze–thaw cycles depend on the lesion. After cryotherapy, a moist wound usually develops, which may become ulcerated, with subsequent crusting and scab formation. After the wound has healed completely, an area of altered pigmentation or frank scarring may remain.

Curettage and electrosurgery. A curette has an oval or cup-shaped component with a cutting edge and a handle. The original curette was developed in the late 1800s; over the years it has proved an invaluable tool for the dermatologist.

When combined with electrosurgery, the curette is an effective treatment for superficial and nodular basal cell carcinoma (BCC) and for squamous cell carcinoma (SCC) in situ.

The two types of electrosurgical technique are:
- electrodesiccation
- electrocautery.

In electrodesiccation, a monoterminal provides a high voltage and low amperage, both of which are superficially destructive to the skin. This technique differs from electrocautery, in which a biterminal supplies a low voltage and high amperage, producing a more deeply destructive effect on the skin.

Although there have been no studies comparing the two, curettage is usually combined with electrodesiccation rather than electrocautery. Because electrodesiccation is only superficially destructive, in combination with curettage it is considered to result in reduced scarring and improved cosmesis, and to make treatment of recurrences easier.

Although there is some variation in the technique of curettage and electrosurgery, the general principles are consistent.

Curettage. After the initial injection of local anesthetic, the tumor is debulked with a medium- or large-sized curette. This is repeatedly drawn through the tumor, including its base. A smaller curette is then used for the margins to ensure the removal of the maximal number of tumor cells. After the neoplasm has been removed, there is a change in tissue consistency – the coarse resistance of normal tissue can be distinguished.

'Saucerization curettage' refers to removal of the tumor in one pass to create a deep saucer-shaped wound.

Electrodesiccation is applied to the base and to an extra 2 mm beyond the rim after satisfactory curettage. This procedure is then repeated. Two or three passes of curettage and electrodesiccation are thought to be adequate for treating non-melanoma skin cancer. One, more superficial, pass suffices for an actinic keratosis.

Outcome. The resulting wounds heal by secondary intention over a 6-week period. Potential side effects include atrophic or hypertrophic scarring, tissue contraction and altered pigmentation at the scar site. Overall, though, this is a safe and effective treatment for many non-melanoma cutaneous malignancies.

Micrographic surgery was developed in the 1940s by Frederick Mohs. The technique relies on the fundamental principle that when a tumor is removed with histological margin control, maximal confidence in the completeness of the excision can be combined with minimal loss of surrounding normal tissue. Mohs' original procedure involved removing the tumor, fixing the tissue and then sectioning the excision margins to reach any tumor involvement. He had excellent cure rates. Today, his technique has been modified: tissue is generally frozen immediately and sectioned, curtailing the length of the procedure (Figure 4.1).

The excised tissue sections and the surgical sites are carefully labeled and oriented so that, following histological examination, the potential locations of residual tumor can be identified. Further sections are then taken according to the histological findings, and the process is repeated until the surgeon is satisfied that the lesion has been excised completely. At this point, surgical repair of the wound can start (Figure 4.2). Mohs micrographic surgery is usually performed under local anesthesia; excision and reconstruction are typically completed in a single day.

The procedure is generally reserved for tumors with aggressive histology that:

- occur at critical anatomic sites on the 'mask' or 'H-zone' of the face, hands or genitals, and
- are larger than 1 cm on the face or 2 cm on the body, and
- have recurred or occur in immunocompromised patients.

'Appropriate use criteria' for Mohs surgery were created in 2012 by the American Academy of Dermatology in collaboration with the

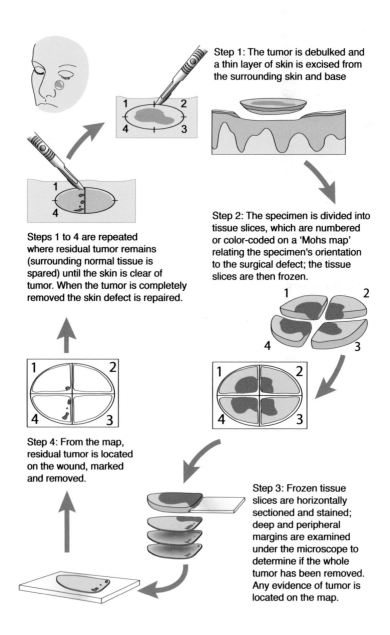

Step 1: The tumor is debulked and a thin layer of skin is excised from the surrounding skin and base

Step 2: The specimen is divided into tissue slices, which are numbered or color-coded on a 'Mohs map' relating the specimen's orientation to the surgical defect; the tissue slices are then frozen.

Steps 1 to 4 are repeated where residual tumor remains (surrounding normal tissue is spared) until the skin is clear of tumor. When the tumor is completely removed the skin defect is repaired.

Step 4: From the map, residual tumor is located on the wound, marked and removed.

Step 3: Frozen tissue slices are horizontally sectioned and stained; deep and peripheral margins are examined under the microscope to determine if the whole tumor has been removed. Any evidence of tumor is located on the map.

Figure 4.1 The steps of Mohs micrographic surgery.

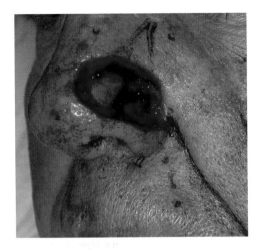

Figure 4.2 Mohs micrographic surgery, in which the tumor has been completely excised and reconstruction can begin.

American College of Mohs Surgery, the American Society for Dermatologic Surgery Association and the American Society for Mohs Surgery. These criteria are based on tumor and patient characteristics and are defined for a variety of scenarios involving BCC, SCC, lentigo maligna, melanoma in situ and rare cutaneous malignancies. Criteria were defined for the average patient; the use of Mohs surgery in individual cases should still be determined by the treating physician.

Photodynamic therapy has proved to be an effective treatment for some non-melanoma skin cancers. The technique involves activating a tissue-localized photosensitizer with visible light. The topical agent and disease-specific irradiance to achieve optimal cell damage and cell death are yet to be established. Patients usually have a histological diagnosis before treatment is started.

In cutaneous PDT with topical 5-aminolevulinic acid (5-ALA), which is licensed in the USA for the treatment of actinic keratosis, the agent is applied to lesions for 1–18 hours, with or without occlusion. It appears to be taken up selectively by and/or retained in diseased tissue during this period and converted to the photosensitizer protoporphyrin IX. The lesion is then illuminated with a laser or incoherent light source within the visible spectrum, with wavelengths in the Soret band (400–410 nm, blue light) being the most effective at triggering the photodynamic reaction.

A number of derivatives of 5-ALA have been synthesized to develop compounds that penetrate the plasma membrane of the target cells and diffuse through epidermal layers more easily. Methyl aminolevulinate (MAL), an ester of ALA, is more lipophilic than free ALA and penetrates more effectively through cutaneous tissue. In an optimal regimen, MAL, 160 mg/g, is applied for 3 hours under an occlusive dressing before illumination with red light (570–670 nm).

PDT can be painful and produces a dose-dependent phototoxicity reaction (erythema and edema) that lasts several days. Otherwise, it has relatively few side effects, and the final cosmesis appears to be good.

Lasers can be used for destruction of precancerous lesions and established non-melanoma skin cancer.

Radiotherapy is a well-established treatment for cutaneous malignancies. Skin cancer is generally treated with conventional radiotherapy using X-rays, which are more penetrating and have a shorter wavelength than both visible and ultraviolet (UV) radiation.

Suspicious lesions are biopsied and a histological diagnosis is confirmed before radiotherapy. The degree to which radiotherapy is employed for skin cancer therapy varies between centers.

Radiosensitive neoplasms include BCC, SCC and some vascular tumors. However, radiotherapy is not as effective for melanoma. Radiotherapy is particularly useful for large neoplasms and those located on the ears, nose and lower eyelid. It is best avoided on the lower legs, at sites subject to repeated trauma and on skin overlying susceptible organs such as the thyroid.

Radiotherapy is a valuable option for the frail elderly, but in younger patients the long-term side effects of skin atrophy, scarring and telangiectasia can make the results cosmetically inferior to those achieved with surgery. In addition, because X-rays are themselves carcinogenic, there is a risk of eventual therapy-induced cancer. Finally, previous radiotherapy makes subsequent surgery more challenging. For this reason, the National Comprehensive Cancer Network recommends radiotherapy for tumors that are not candidates for surgical excision.

Management of at-risk patients

It is important to identify those individuals who are at high risk of cutaneous malignancies so that management strategies can be implemented. Management strategies are needed for patients with:

- benign lesions that may become malignant
- premalignant lesions
- substantial previous UV radiation exposure/chronic photodamage
- immunosuppression
- a genetic predisposition for cutaneous malignancies.

Benign lesions

Congenital melanocytic nevi (CMN). The management of CMN is not well defined and should be individualized. Excision of giant nevi is often not feasible, but, if performed, should take place early in life. This may require staged surgery with tissue expansion. There is no evidence that prophylactic excision of CMN reduces the risk of melanoma. The primary melanoma may not develop within the CMN and there are cases of melanoma developing under a previously excised area. Surgery is often offered to patients with giant CMN for aesthetic reasons if there is facial involvement or for physically troublesome areas like large nodules. In addition, any suspicious atypical areas should be excised for pathological investigation. It is not usual practice to excise all small- and medium-sized CMN (see Figures 3.15–3.17).

British guidelines recommend lifelong monitoring by a specialist for patients with giant CMN. In addition, all those with medium-sized or giant CMN require education on self-examination and the need for periodic photographic surveillance.

Individuals with satellite nevi or large CMN are at increased risk of neurological abnormalities, including neurocutaneous melanosis. This excessive proliferation of melanocytes within the CNS can be identified with MRI. Experts recommend neurodevelopmental assessments in early childhood for those with giant CMN or satellite lesions, as most neurological complications occur within the first 2 years of life. There is value in performing gadolinium-enhanced MRI of the CNS in infants under 6 months of age who are born with satellite lesions. These children are most at risk, and if radiological abnormalities are identified they require management under the care of pediatric neurologists.

Self-examination. Patients should be advised to carry out self-examination monthly in front of a full-length mirror in a room with plenty of light (Figure 4.3). A hand-held mirror is useful for viewing areas out of plain sight, or a relative or close friend can help examine those hard-to-see areas like the lower back, back of the thighs or scalp. On the first examination, the patient should study the entire surface of their skin carefully to learn the usual look and feel of moles, blemishes, freckles and other marks, and the patterns they make. Ask patients to contact you if they notice any changes over time (e.g. in size, shape, color or feel), or find anything unusual.

Atypical nevus syndrome. The presence of atypical nevi is a significant risk factor for melanoma (see Figures 3.19–3.21). The risk is lower in a patient with only one or two atypical moles and no family history of melanoma than in a patient who has both atypical nevi and a family history of atypical nevi and melanoma (familial atypical mole and melanoma syndrome). The term 'atypical nevus syndrome' is used to represent this spectrum of phenotypic expression.

Individuals with atypical nevi should be encouraged to self-examine every 1–3 months to look for changes in their moles. Surveillance of their nevi by a doctor is also recommended and can be aided by cutaneous photographs. The importance of protection from the sun must be emphasized and family members should also be screened.

Spitz nevus. The optimal management of a Spitz nevus is not clearly defined. Although the nevus is benign (see Figure 3.5), it can be difficult to exclude melanoma definitively. For this reason, an excisional biopsy with re-excision of any positive margins is the treatment of choice.

Genetic predisposition and other 'at-risk' factors
Genetic counseling should be offered to individuals with nevoid BCC syndrome, xeroderma pigmentosum and the xeroderma pigmentosum variants.

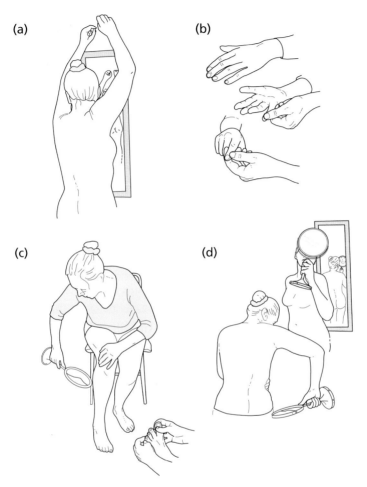

Figure 4.3 Self-examination advice for patients: (a) Standing in front of a full-length mirror, check your face, neck, ears, chest and stomach. Look at both the front and back of your body in the mirror. Then raise your arms and look at your left and right sides. Women should lift their breasts to check the skin underneath. Also, use a hand mirror while in front of the full-length mirror to check the back of your neck, shoulders and upper arms. (b) Check both sides of your arms, both sides of your hands and your fingernails. (c) Sitting down, check your legs, including the back of your calves and thighs, the bottom of your feet, the spaces between your toes and your toenails. (d) Using a hand mirror, inspect your lower back, buttocks, legs and genital area.

Xeroderma pigmentosum. Patients are managed with strict photoprotection, including sun avoidance, a daily sunscreen, self-examination and regular surveillance by their dermatologist. Oral retinoids such as isotretinoin or acitretin have a prophylactic role.

Nevoid basal cell carcinoma syndrome (Gorlin's syndrome). Individuals require vigilant dermatological surveillance (see Figures 3.32–3.33). Early diagnosis is advantageous so that strict photoprotective measures can be instituted from a young age. However, as a high rate of disease arises from spontaneous mutations, early diagnosis can be difficult. Treatment of BCC is similar to that for BCC in an unaffected individual, except that radiotherapy is avoided.

Immunosuppression. Cutaneous malignancies associated with iatrogenic immunosuppression and HIV infection can be atypical and aggressive (Figure 4.4). A high index of suspicion is required when examining immunocompromised patients, with a low threshold for skin biopsies. In addition, this population requires regular skin surveillance and education about strict sun protection.

Albinism describes a range of genetic conditions characterized by loss of pigment in the hair, skin and eyes. Patients with albinism may have no, or very little, pigmentation in their skin and are at high risk for skin cancer due to the absence of protective melanin.

Substantial ultraviolet radiation exposure. Individuals who have received a large cumulative dose of UV radiation or episodic UV

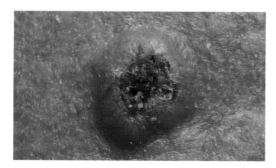

Figure 4.4 Squamous cell carcinoma in an organ-transplant recipient.

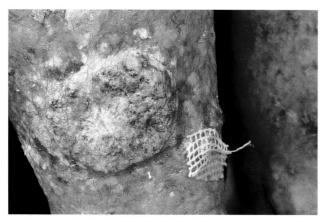

Figure 4.5 Squamous cell carcinoma associated with excessive sunbed use.

radiation burns are at increased risk of skin cancer. If there is a history of severe sunburn, significant sun exposure or sunbed use (Figure 4.5), the patient should be offered education on sun protection and self-examination. A standard measure of the skin's response to UV radiation is the Fitzpatrick skin type, which evaluates patient-reported sensitivity to UV radiation (Table 4.1). Patients with a tendency to burn (types I–III) are at higher risk for skin cancer and should be educated accordingly.

TABLE 4.1

Fitzpatrick classification of skin type

Fitzpatrick skin phototype	Sunburn tendency	Suntan tendency
I	Always burns easily	Never tans
II	Always burns easily	Tans slightly
III	Burns moderately	Tans gradually
IV	Burns minimally	Tans moderately
V	Rarely burns	Tans profusely
VI	Never burns	Tans profusely

Premalignant lesions

Actinic keratosis (see Figures 3.10–3.12). Topical treatment options include imiquimod, 5-fluorouracil, ingenol mebutate and diclofenac sodium. Other procedures include cryotherapy, PDT and curettage and/or electrocautery. Topical therapies are particularly valuable for the treatment of diffuse and multiple actinic keratoses. They can be used to treat field change where numerous actinic keratoses are evident within an area of sun-damaged skin. These fields are thought to be at increased risk of transformation to squamous cell carcinoma. PDT and surgical procedures may be offered to patients with hyperkeratotic or only a few discrete actinic keratoses.

Imiquimod is available at 5% and 3.75% strengths in the UK (also 2.5% in the USA). It is an immunomodulatory agent for the treatment of actinic keratoses. The 5% formulation may also be used to treat small superficial BCCs. Imiquimod and other imidazoquinolones activate antigen-presenting cells, inducing secretion of proinflammatory cytokines. Interferon α, tumor necrosis factor α and interleukin (IL)-12 have a central role in mediating the resultant cytotoxic effect. The 3.75% strength is applied daily for 2 weeks followed by a 2-week treatment break, then further daily application for another 2 weeks. A treatment regimen of three applications a week for 4 weeks has been proposed for the use of 5% imiquimod. The inflammatory reaction varies and may be similar to that seen with 5-fluorouracil (see below). Imiquimod is not recommended for use in immunocompromised patients. The 3.75% formulation may be applied to an area on the scalp or face of up to 200 cm² at a time, effectively treating a large field.

5-fluorouracil cream is available in 5%, 1% and 0.5% strengths. It is an established treatment for actinic keratosis, and the 5% strength is also effective against superficial BCC and in situ SCC. The mode of action is thought to be a direct cytotoxic effect on neoplastic cells. The cream is usually applied once or twice daily for 2–4 weeks. Patients should be counseled to expect erythema, mild discomfort, crusting and oozing. The lesions typically heal over a 2-week period following discontinuation of treatment.

Ingenol mebutate is a novel agent extracted from the petty spurge plant *Euphorbia peplus*. It activates protein kinase C, generating a neutrophilic reaction. Available at 0.015% strength for the face and scalp and 0.05% for the body, ingenol mebutate is approved in the USA, Australia, UK and other European countries for the treatment of actinic keratoses. It is applied daily for 3 days on the face and scalp or 2 days on the body. The resulting inflammation is similar to that seen with other topical agents, although the brief duration of treatment results in faster overall resolution, improving patient adherence. Ingenol mebutate has not been tested in immunocompromised patients.

3% diclofenac sodium gel is a non-steroidal anti-inflammatory drug (NSAID), licensed in the USA and UK for the treatment of actinic keratosis. It is applied to the area twice daily for 60–90 days. This medication is favored for long-term use against mild actinic keratoses; it causes a mild level of erythema and crusting. Although generally well tolerated, this preparation is contraindicated in those with an allergy to NSAIDs.

Cryotherapy. Normally, actinic keratoses respond to a single freeze–thaw cycle with a freezing time of 5–15 seconds. This is an excellent in-office therapy for a small number of actinic keratoses, but is less effective for broad fields of actinic damage. There is brief, moderate discomfort during the procedure, and the lesions blister and crust during the following 2 weeks. Treatment that is too aggressive can result in a permanent hypopigmented patch.

Photodynamic therapy is effective for thin and moderate thickness actinic keratoses and achieves a very good cosmetic outcome. MAL PDT is effective in most locations except acral lesions, which respond less well to PDT. 5-ALA PDT is best directed at non-hyperkeratotic actinic keratoses on the face. The treatment is performed in a clinic or physician's office; there is some discomfort and the resulting inflammation is similar to that seen with other topical agents. Most countries recommend an initial single treatment, repeated at 3 months if required.

Curettage and/or electrocautery is used by many dermatologists. It is typically reserved for hypertrophic actinic keratoses resistant to cryotherapy. In some cases, curettage is performed before PDT or topical treatment to enhance penetrance.

Lentigo maligna. If left untreated, a small proportion of cases of lentigo maligna (see Figures 3.22 and 3.23) will progress to lentigo maligna melanoma (see Figure 3.44). Treatment options include conventional surgical excision, Mohs micrographic surgery and topical imiquimod.

The mainstay of treatment is conventional surgical excision with a 5–10 mm surgical margin, though the highest cure rates are seen using Mohs micrographic surgery. Cryotherapy has been used, though there is little evidence to support its use. Success with topical imiquimod has, however, been reported. These two treatments are controversial and should not take the place of complete excision when possible. In elderly patients, particularly those with a large facial lesion where progression is unlikely within their lifespan, radiotherapy or observation of the lentigo maligna may be the most appropriate approach.

Malignant lesions

Basal cell carcinoma. There are a number of effective treatments available for BCC, both surgical and non-surgical. Factors such as the patient's preference, age and health, as well as the clinical and histological subtype, size and site need to be considered when making a management decision (see Figures 3.24–3.31). The non-surgical treatments (radiotherapy, topical 5-fluorouracil, topical imiquimod and PDT) have the disadvantage of not generating a pathological specimen. Therefore, a histological diagnosis cannot be made for patients treated by non-surgical means.

Surgical excision is the most common treatment for primary BCC and is very effective. It is the treatment of choice for most recurrent, nodular, morpheic or superficial facial BCCs, but indications for Mohs micrographic surgery should be absent (see opposite). It is useful to curette the BCC before excision so that the 'naked-eye' tumor margin can be delineated.

The optimal excision margin depends on the BCC subtype and size. For a primary BCC with a diameter of less than 2 cm, there is evidence that a 3-mm surgical excision margin will clear the tumor in 85% of cases, a rate that increases to 95% clearance with a margin of 4–5 mm. The excision margin must be wider for morpheic and large BCCs. Similar studies show that a morpheic BCC excised with a margin of 5 mm has an 82% peripheral clearance rate; however, with a margin of 13–15 mm, the rate improves to over 95% clearance. Recurrent BCCs also have lower cure rates, and excision margins of 5–10 mm have been suggested.

There is controversy over the management of incompletely excised BCC. The tumor does not necessarily have to be totally removed to achieve complete resolution. Studies have shown wide variation in the risk of recurrence, from 16% to 60%. The recurrence rate is high when the deep margins are involved or the lesion is a high-risk BCC.

Mohs micrographic surgery is a labor-intensive specialized procedure (see Figure 4.1) that achieves very high BCC cure rates: 99% 5-year cure rate for primary BCC and 94% for recurrent BCC. This treatment is reserved for aggressive histological BCC subtypes located on critical or high-risk sites. It is not mandated for all BCCs because it is time-consuming and expensive, and the morbidity may exceed the benefit. Table 4.2 lists features of a BCC that should prompt consideration of Mohs micrographic surgery.

Curettage with electrosurgery is a valuable treatment for small well-defined primary BCCs that have a non-aggressive histology and are not located on critical sites; the 5-year cure rate for this treatment has been shown to be as high as 97%. The cure rates are variable and

---

TABLE 4.2

Basal cell carcinoma: indications for Mohs micrographic surgery*

Site	**Histology**
Eyelids	Morpheic
Nose	Infiltrative
Nasolabial folds	Micronodular
Ears	Basosquamous
Lips	Perineural spread
	Perivascular involvement
Size	**Other**
> 2 cm in diameter	Recurrent

*British Association of Dermatologists' guidelines for the management of basal cell carcinoma.

seem to be operator dependent. Studies show overall cure rates to be 92% after 5 years for primary BCC and 60% for recurrent BCC. Curettage and electrosurgery may not be successful for recurrent or morpheic BCC.

Cryosurgery is best reserved for the treatment of extrafacial superficial BCC; in this situation, the cure rates can be high. These lesions require prolonged freezing for 20–30 seconds before the freeze–thaw cycle is repeated. Such prolonged freeze–thaw cycles are associated with significant morbidity.

Radiotherapy has been used to treat cutaneous malignancies for many years. It can be an excellent option for those not wanting to undergo surgery, and has a 5-year cure rate of 91% for primary BCC and 90% for recurrent BCC. It is generally thought that radiotherapy is best used for primary nodular and solid BCC.

Topical 5-fluorouracil is not commonly used to treat BCC, but it can be valuable in the management of superficial BCC, particularly of the face.

Topical imiquimod 5% cream is a well-recognized treatment for small superficial BCC. The standard regimen is imiquimod application to the BCC and adjacent skin five times weekly for a 6-week period.

Photodynamic therapy is an evolving technique. Current evidence confirms 5-ALA PDT and MAL PDT as effective treatments for superficial BCC. MAL PDT is effective for the treatment of nodular BCC, although higher cure rates are achieved with surgical excision. It is also less effective in organ-transplant recipients. Patients typically receive two PDT treatments, with a 7-day interval.

Topical PDT offers good cosmetic results, and MAL PDT is licensed for the treatment of superficial and nodular BCCs in Europe, New Zealand and Australia. PDT is used off label for BCC in the USA.

Hedgehog pathway inhibitors are novel targeted molecular agents that are being developed for rare cases of metastatic tumors and tumors that are so advanced that cure with surgery and radiation is technically impossible without significant morbidity, such as loss of an eye or limb. Vismodegib is the first-in-class systemic agent licensed for metastatic and locally advanced BCC; other agents are currently in clinical trials.

Follow-up. Most patients are reviewed 3–6 months after treatment. For an uncomplicated BCC, ongoing specialist care is not required. However, patients are advised to see their family doctor every 6–12 months so that any recurrence or a further tumor at another site can be detected.

In situ squamous cell carcinoma. Treatments reflect the range of clinical disease encountered. Bowen's disease is the most common form of in situ SCC and a number of acceptable treatments are available. There are few studies comparing the efficacy of different treatment options, but expert opinion is that no single approach is best for all clinical situations.

The treatments discussed below have similar recurrence rates. In addition, preliminary studies have shown laser therapy and topical imiquimod to be effective. The optimal regimen for imiquimod application has not yet been determined.

It is not uncommon for Bowen's disease to develop on the lower leg (see Figure 3.37), which is a site of poor healing.

Cryotherapy is a useful tool in the treatment of Bowen's disease. However, it can be painful and healing may be prolonged. Although there is some controversy regarding the best regimen, a single 30-second freeze–thaw cycle appears to be as effective as two 30-second freeze–thaw cycles. Treatment with two freeze–thaw cycles of 20 seconds has demonstrated efficacy, but a single 15-second freeze–thaw cycle is generally considered to give inferior results.

Curettage with electrosurgery usually results in a less severe wound than that produced by cryotherapy. It can also be an effective treatment for Bowen's disease, though studies report cure rates ranging from 27% to 98%. The reasons for this variability are not clear and may relate to physician technique.

Surgical excision is often used, depending on the size and site of the lesion. Mohs micrographic surgery is recommended for digital and subungual Bowen's disease.

Photodynamic therapy is an effective treatment for Bowen's disease, and appears to offer good cosmesis and limited adverse effects. It is of particular value for large or multiple lesions and for sites of poor healing. PDT is used off label for Bowen's disease in the USA.

Topical 5-fluorouracil is usually applied once or twice daily to the in situ SCC for between 1 week and 2 months. It is a useful treatment for extragenital Bowen's disease, and penile and anal intraepithelial neoplasia (see Figure 3.39).

Radiotherapy. Although radiotherapy boasts high cure rates, it is often not a first-line treatment because there can be complications with poor wound healing.

Follow-up. Of the in situ SCC subtypes, perianal Bowen's disease has the highest recurrence rate. Patients require long-term specialist follow-up because they are at risk of further in situ SCC and invasive perianal SCC. Perianal Bowen's disease may be associated with high-risk human papillomavirus (HPV) infection; for this reason, referral to gynecology or colorectal surgery is recommended for internal evaluation.

Keratoacanthoma (see Figures 3.13, 3.14 and 3.36). Treatment options include:

• surgical excision
• curettage and electrosurgery
• Mohs micrographic surgery.

As it is difficult to differentiate keratoacanthoma from invasive SCC (see pages 48–9 and 52–4 and Figure 3.14), both clinically and histologically, it is prudent to use SCC treatments for these lesions. Keratoacanthoma is therefore most commonly excised surgically, but curettage and electrosurgery may be appropriate for small classic lesions. In select cases, intralesional injection with 5-fluorouracil is used.

Keratoacanthoma developing on the central face is characteristically more aggressive and Mohs micrographic surgery warrants consideration.

Invasive squamous cell carcinoma. It is necessary to extirpate invasive SCC completely because of its potential to metastasize. This neoplasm usually spreads initially to the local lymph nodes via the lymphatics. SCC also has a tendency to develop in-transit metastases: these are cutaneous tumors adjacent to, but not contiguous with, the primary SCC.

Factors associated with high-risk SCC include large size, recurrent tumor and poor differentiation, as well as development at sites such as non-sun-exposed regions, an ear, a lip, or an area of skin damage or inflammation (see Figures 3.40 and 3.41). Patients with high-risk neoplasms are ideally managed by a multidisciplinary team of dermatologists, cutaneous surgeons and oncologists.

Surgical excision is the treatment of choice for invasive SCC in most patients. It achieves good cure rates, and enables the SCC to be fully characterized histopathologically and the adequacy of the treatment to be verified microscopically.

For a well-defined low-risk SCC with diameter less than 2 cm, excision with a minimum of a 4-mm margin is sufficient and provides a 95% cure rate. A wider margin of 6 mm or more may be required for high-risk SCC. This excision margin may be smaller if the SCC is excised with Mohs micrographic surgery or if there is intraoperative histological examination of the specimen edges. A wider margin is required because a high-risk cutaneous SCC may have surrounding microscopic in-transit metastases that must be removed. In addition, larger tumors have a greater degree of microscopic tumor extension.

Mohs micrographic surgery (see Figure 4.1) should be considered for high-risk and recurrent SCC, particularly tumors at sites where it is difficult to achieve adequate excision margins. With reportedly the best cure rates for high-risk SCC, this is probably the treatment of choice for this subgroup.

Curettage with electrosurgery should be restricted to the treatment of small (< 10 mm diameter) well-differentiated primary SCC. High cure rates have been reported. Recommendations on the use of this treatment differ. It is not recommended for SCC treatment in the USA but, conversely, it has a role in SCC management in the UK, where it is included in SCC guidelines. With this technique, it is difficult to ascertain histologically whether the tumor has been removed completely.

Radiotherapy achieves cure rates comparable with those achieved using other treatments. It is the first-line treatment for non-resectable tumors for which the morbidity from surgery is considered too high. Radiotherapy is not suitable when the tumor has indistinct margins.

Management of nodal metastasis. If local lymph nodes are enlarged, they should be sampled by fine-needle aspiration or excisional biopsy for histological assessment. Ideally, node-positive patients should be reviewed in a multidisciplinary setting. Metastatic lymph node disease is usually treated with regional lymph node dissection. The use of imaging for nodal staging is controversial, and there are no guidelines for imaging. Physicians may elect to image high-risk SCC to evaluate for nodal or perineural metastasis. There is no strong evidence to favor sentinel lymph node biopsy or prophylactic elective lymph node dissection.

Follow-up. The patient with a treated high-risk invasive SCC is best observed every 6 months for 5 years. The specialist, family doctor or patient can perform the surveillance. In addition, early detection and treatment of recurrent SCC has been shown to improve survival. Therefore, patients should be educated on self-examination of the surgical scar site, local skin and lymph nodes. They should be educated to look for new or changing pigmentation, nodularity or ulceration.

Melanoma. The definitive treatment of primary cutaneous melanoma (see Figures 3.46 and 3.47) is surgical excision. After the diagnosis has been confirmed by excisional biopsy, surgical re-excision is usually performed.

Surgical excision. The recommended excision margins are 0.5 cm, with excision to subcutaneous fat for melanoma in situ and 1–3 cm with excision to fascia for invasive melanoma. The rationale for removing a portion of normal skin surrounding the visible lesion is to prevent local recurrence. Melanoma cells have the capacity to migrate locally from the original tumor. For this reason, Mohs surgery is not recommended for invasive melanoma. Recommendations for the width of margins for surgical excision based on the Breslow thickness of the melanoma are presented in Table 4.3.

The margins should be measured clinically at the time of surgery and should not be imposed retrospectively following the histology report on the margin of excision, nor used erroneously to justify

further surgery. There are circumstances in which the recommended

TABLE 4.3

Recommended excision margins for primary melanoma

Breslow thickness of melanoma	UK guideline margins	NCCN guideline margins	Australia/ New Zealand guideline margins
Lentigo maligna and in situ melanoma	5 mm to achieve complete excision	5 mm	5 mm
< 1 mm	1 cm	1 cm	1 cm
1–2 mm	1–2 cm	1–2 cm	1–2 cm
2–4 mm	2–3 cm	2 cm	1–2 cm (preferable to take 2 cm)
> 4 mm	3 cm	2 cm	2 cm

NCCN, National Comprehensive Cancer Network.

margins may not be technically achievable or cosmetically or functionally desirable, but these decisions should be made by experts and fully explained to the patient. If there is already evidence of metastatic disease, radical re-excision is illogical.

The treatment of lentigo maligna melanoma may be difficult because the margins can be clinically and histologically indeterminate (see Figure 3.44). As a minimum, the nodular component of the lentigo maligna melanoma should be excised with the recommended margins. In some cases, wide margin excision of lentigo maligna melanoma is followed by Mohs surgery to establish peripheral margins before reconstruction.

Management of lymph node disease. If there is clinical or radiological suspicion of lymph node involvement, fine-needle aspiration of the relevant nodes is recommended. It may be necessary to perform an open biopsy if there is persistent lymphadenopathy and fine-needle aspiration is negative.

Lymph node metastases are treated with radical lymph node dissection. Elective lymph node dissection has not been shown to be advantageous for patients where there is no evidence of nodal involvement.

Sentinel lymph node biopsy. There is controversy over the role of intraoperative lymphatic mapping and biopsy of sentinel lymph nodes. The technique was first described by Morton in 1992 and is usually performed at the time of the wider re-excision. The sentinel lymph node is the first node in the lymphatic basin that drains the primary melanoma. It is dissected after identification by lymphoscintigraphy. If histological examination proves metastatic involvement of the sentinel lymph node, the patient undergoes complete nodal dissection. Sentinel lymph node biopsy is a sensitive tool for staging and prognosis, but it is not therapeutic. The controversy surrounding this arises because a positive result with associated lymph node dissection does not improve patient outcomes or alter subsequent management. In research settings, sentinel lymph node biopsy is most often performed in patients with intermediate thickness melanoma (1–4 mm). The reported complication rates for this procedure are 5–10%; however, these rates increase to 20–40% for those who subsequently undergo complete lymph node dissection. It is also important that patients are aware that there is a false-negative rate of up to 25%. Further trials are required to clarify the role of sentinel lymph node biopsy.

Systemic therapy. Once melanoma has spread beyond the regional lymph nodes, it is the leading cause of skin cancer death. Until recently, chemotherapy was the standard of care for stage IV non-resectable melanoma. More recent advances in immunotherapy include interferon α-2b, granulocyte-macrophage colony-stimulating factor (GM-CSF), IL-12 and anti-cytotoxic T lymphocyte antigen 4 (CTLA-4) antibodies. Newer molecular therapies target specific proteins in signaling pathways, such as the serine/threonine protein kinase BRAF, MAPK/ERK kinase (MEK) and phosphoinositide 3-kinase (PI3K). These treatments are best prescribed by oncologists.

Follow-up. There is no evidence to justify a specific follow-up interval, therefore follow-up regimens differ between countries. Follow-up should provide an opportunity for patient education and support in addition to detection of recurrence or further primary melanoma.

The US guidelines sensibly suggest that follow-up be determined on a case-by-case basis with reference to individual factors that include:

- Breslow thickness
- number of melanomas
- presence and number of atypical nevi
- family history
- anxiety
- patient capability.

British guidelines recommend that patients with stage IA melanoma be followed up at 3-monthly to 6-monthly intervals for the first year and then discharged. For stage IB to IIC melanoma, they suggest 3-monthly review for 3 years followed by 6-monthly follow-up for a further 2 years. In this group, the risk of recurrence is greatest at 2–4 years after the primary excision. Those with stage IIIA disease are followed up with this same regimen; most of these patients will have had complete lymphadenectomy following the positive sentinel lymph node biopsy. Finally, for stage IIIB to resected IV melanoma, they recommend 3-monthly review for 3 years then 6-monthly review for 2 years followed by annual review for a further 5 years.

The Australian and New Zealand melanoma guidelines propose another follow-up regimen. Their recommendation is for 6-monthly follow-up intervals for 5 years, then ongoing annual review for stage I disease. In many patients with stage I disease, the need for follow-up is dictated more by the patient's risk of having a second melanoma than by the risk of relapse from the original. For patients with stage II or III disease, 3- or 4-monthly appointments for 5 years followed by ongoing annual review is the recommended follow-up schedule.

At follow-up, symptoms should be sought, the scar and the rest of the skin examined, and lymphadenopathy and organomegaly excluded clinically. Patient self-examination should be encouraged. Investigations are not necessary unless clinically indicated.

Key points – management

- Excisional surgery is the gold standard for the treatment of most established skin cancers.
- Cryotherapy is the gold standard for the treatment of actinic keratosis.
- A number of non-surgical therapies are effective for the treatment of premalignant non-melanoma skin cancer and low-grade basal cell carcinomas (BCCs).
- Mohs micrographic surgery is the gold standard for selected BCCs.

Key references

Ahmed I, Berth-Jones J. Imiquimod: a novel treatment for lentigo maligna. *Br J Dermatol* 2000; 143:843–5.

Australian Cancer Network Melanoma Guidelines Revision Working Party. *Clinical Practice Guidelines for the Management of Melanoma in Australia and New Zealand*. Wellington: Cancer Council Australia and Australian Cancer Network, Sydney and New Zealand Guidelines Group, 2008. Available at www.nhmrc.gov.au/_files_nhmrc/publications/attachments/cp111.pdf, last accessed 19 August 2013.

Bunker CB. Scientific evidence and expert clinical opinion for the investigation and management of stage I malignant melanoma. In: MacKie RM, Murray D, Rosin RD et al, eds. *The Effective Management of Malignant Melanoma*. London: Aesculapius Medical Press, 2001: 37–44.

Chong K, Daud A, Ortiz-Urda S, Arron ST. Cutting edge in medical management of cutaneous oncology. *Semin Cutan Med Surg* 2012;31: 140–9.

Connolly SM, Baker DR, Coldiron BM et al. AAD/ACMS/ASDSA/ASMS 2012 appropriate use criteria for Mohs micrographic surgery: a report of the American Academy of Dermatology, American College of Mohs Surgery, American Society for Dermatologic Surgery Association, and the American Society for Mohs Surgery. *J Am Acad Dermatol* 2012;67:531–50.

Cox NH, Eedy DJ, Morton CA. Guidelines for management of Bowen's disease: 2006 update. *Br J Dermatol* 2007;156:11–21.

Geisse JK, Rich P, Pandya A et al. Imiquimod 5% cream for the treatment of superficial basal cell carcinoma: a double-blind, randomized, vehicle-controlled study. *J Am Acad Dermatol* 2002;47:390–8.

Graham GF. Cryosurgery in the management of cutaneous malignancies. *Clin Dermatol* 2001;19:321–7.

Kinsler VA, Chong WK, Aylett SE, Atherton DJ. Complications of congenital melanocytic naevi in children: analysis of 16 years' experience and clinical practice. *Br J Dermatol* 2008;159:907–14.

Marsden JR, Newton-Bishop JA, Burrows L et al. Revised U.K. guidelines for the management of cutaneous melanoma 2010. *Br J Dermatol* 2010;163:238–56.

Morton CA, McKenna KE, Rhodes LE. Guidelines for topical photodynamic therapy: update. *Br J Dermatol* 2008;159:1245–66.

Motley R, Kersey P, Lawrence C. Multiprofessional guidelines for the management of the patient with primary cutaneous squamous cell carcinoma. *Br J Dermatol* 2002;146:18–25.

Primary Care Dermatology Society. Actinic keratosis (syn. solar keratosis). Management. www.pcds.org.uk/clinical-guidance/actinic-keratosis-syn.-solar-keratosis#management

Sekulic A, Migden MR, Oro AE et al. Efficacy and safety of vismodegib in advanced basal-cell carcinoma. *N Engl J Med* 2012;366:2171–9.

Sheridan AT, Dawber RPR. Curettage, electrosurgery and skin cancer. *Australas J Dermatol* 2000;41:19–30.

Sober AJ, Chuang TY, Duvic M et al. Guidelines of care for primary cutaneous melanoma. *J Am Acad Dermatol* 2001;45:579–86.

Stockfleth E, Gupta G, Perkis K et al. Reduction in lesions from Lmax: a new concept for assessing efficacy of field-directed therapy for actinic keratosis. Results with imiquimod 3.75%. *Eur J Dermatol* 2014;24:23–7.

Stockfleth E, Meyer T, Benninghoff B et al. A randomized, double-blind, vehicle-controlled study to assess 5% imiquimod cream for the treatment of multiple actinic keratoses. *Arch Dermatol* 2002;138:1498–502.

Telfer NR, Colver GB, Morton CA. Guidelines for the management of basal cell carcinoma. *Br J Dermatol* 2008;159:35–48.

Wong SL, Balch CM, Hurley P et al. Sentinel lymph node biopsy for melanoma: American Society of Clinical Oncology and Society of Surgical Oncology joint clinical practice guideline. *J Clin Oncol* 2012;30:2912–18.

Basal cell carcinoma

The patient with a treated uncomplicated basal cell carcinoma (BCC) can expect an excellent outcome. Following appropriate treatment, the recurrence rate is less than 10%. Factors associated with poor prognosis include:

- infiltrative, morpheic or basosquamous histological subtypes
- histological evidence of perivascular or perineural involvement
- immunocompromised status
- large or recurrent BCC
- location on the ear, nose, nasolabial fold or eyelid.

The literature suggests that, of recurrent BCC, 33%, 50% and 66% reappear within 1, 2 and 3 years of treatment, respectively. In addition, once an individual has developed one BCC they have a greater risk of developing further BCC than those with no history of this tumor.

BCC spreads slowly by direct extension of the primary tumor (Figure 5.1). The morbidity from this neoplasm is largely caused by the destruction of surrounding normal tissue. This neoplasm very rarely metastasizes. The BCCs that appear to have greatest metastatic potential are the deeply invasive morpheic tumors of the face or scalp.

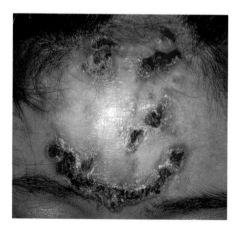

Figure 5.1 Recurrent basal cell carcinoma on the forehead.

Squamous cell carcinoma

In situ squamous cell carcinoma. The recurrence rate following treatment for extragenital Bowen's disease is 5–10%. If left untreated, approximately 3% of extragenital in situ squamous cell carcinomas (SCCs) will progress to invasive SCC, and the risk is higher with anogenital involvement.

An apparent relationship between Bowen's disease and internal malignancy was reported in the 1950s. A subsequent meta-analysis concluded that there was no significant association.

Invasive squamous cell carcinoma. If the invasive SCC is identified and treated early, the prognosis is better. The factors affecting tumor recurrence and metastatic potential are listed in Table 5.1.

Metastases are most likely to develop from larger fast-growing poorly differentiated SCCs and those arising at high-risk sites. If the

TABLE 5.1

Risk factors for recurrence and metastasis of squamous cell carcinoma

Histological features	Dimensions
Poorly differentiated	Diameter > 20 mm
Perineural involvement	Depth > 4 mm or extending into the subcutaneous fat
Vascular or lymphatic invasion	
Desmoplastic, spindle or acantholytic subtypes	
Location	**Host factors**
Lip	Immunosuppression
Ear	
Non-sun-exposed sites	
Sites of scarring, Bowen's disease, chronic ulceration or inflammation	
Other	
Recurrent	

diameter of the SCC is greater than 20 mm, there is a 15% risk of recurrence and a 30% risk of metastasis. By comparison, the rates for smaller lesions are 7% and 9%, respectively. Neoplasms that extend into subcutaneous tissue and those with a depth greater than 4 mm also have a poor prognosis – 45% of these will metastasize.

At the time of initial therapy, incompletely excised and recurrent SCC is more likely to metastasize than primary SCC.

The method of treatment influences the outcome. Recurrence rates following Mohs micrographic surgery have been shown to be significantly lower than those seen with other treatment methods. One meta-analysis reported a local recurrence rate of 3.1% with Mohs micrographic surgery compared with 10.9% with non-Mohs techniques for primary SCC of the skin or lip.

Virtually all SCC recurrences and metastases occur within 5 years of initial therapy.

Melanoma

In situ melanoma does not have metastatic potential, though there may be local recurrence. Approximately 5% of lentigo maligna recur within 2 years of treatment. Cure rates approach 100% with Mohs micrographic surgery and this treatment modality should be considered for recurrent lentigo maligna. In situ melanomas of acral and genital skin have a higher rate of local recurrence.

Of the known prognostic variables for melanoma, Breslow thickness is the strongest predictor of survival. Why Breslow thickness is such a powerful prognostic factor is not known – it may be that it reflects tumor volume. However, the measurement is not precise, and human variability and error need to be taken into account. The prognosis with reference to the Breslow thickness is presented in Table 5.2.

Other histological variables that adversely influence prognosis include:

- melanoma ulceration
- Clark's level of invasion (see Glossary, page 4)
- numerous mitoses
- tumor regression

TABLE 5.2

Melanoma: approximate 5-year survival rates in relation to Breslow thickness

Breslow thickness	Survival
In situ	95–100%
< 1 mm	95–100%
1–2 mm	80–96%
2–4 mm	60–75%
> 4 mm	50%

- perineural infiltration
- vascular or lymphatic invasion
- the presence of microsatellites.

Sentinel lymph node biopsy has prognostic value. If the melanoma Breslow thickness is between 1.2 mm and 3.5 mm and sentinel lymph node biopsy is positive, then the patient's 5-year survival rate is 75% compared with 90% if the sentinel lymph node biopsy is negative.

Lesions located on the extremities have a better outcome than axial lesions, and there is a survival advantage for women and for patients aged under 50.

Neither pregnancy nor hormone replacement therapy has been shown to influence prognosis. Placental and fetal metastases are possible in stage IV disease.

If the patient presents with melanoma and regional nodal metastasis, then the presence of tumor ulceration has greater prognostic value than the Breslow thickness. In this group, the number of metastatic lymph nodes and the magnitude of tumor burden are also significant predictors of outcome.

Survival rates for melanoma stages I, II and III are shown in Table 5.3.

Although melanoma can metastasize widely, metastatic deposits most frequently occur in the skin (Figure 5.2), soft tissues, lung and liver. Recent advances in melanoma therapies have demonstrated significant survival benefits for patients with metastatic disease. Prior

TABLE 5.3

Melanoma survival rates in primary tumor and regional lymph node disease*

Stage	Characteristics of primary tumor (including Breslow thickness)	Survival at 5 years
IA	$\leq$ 1.0 mm, no ulceration and mitoses < 1/mm^2	97%
IB	$\leq$ 1.0 mm with ulceration or mitoses $\geq$ 1/mm^2	94%
	1.01–2.0 mm, no ulceration	91%
IIA	1.01–2.0 mm with ulceration	82%
	2.01–4.0 mm, no ulceration	79%
IIB	2.01–4.0 mm with ulceration	68%
	> 4.0 mm, no ulceration	71%
IIC	> 4.0 mm with ulceration	53%
IIIA	Any thickness, no ulceration and nodal micrometastases	78%
IIIB	Any thickness with ulceration and nodal micrometastases Any thickness, no ulceration and $\leq$ 3 palpable nodes Any thickness, no ulceration or nodes but in-transit or satellite metastasis/metastases	59%
IIIC	Any thickness with ulceration and $\leq$ 3 palpable nodes Any thickness $\pm$ ulceration and $\geq$ 4 palpable nodes or matted nodes or nodes and in-transit metastases Any thickness with ulceration and no nodes but in-transit or satellite metastasis/metastases	40%

Adapted from Edge SB et al. 2010.

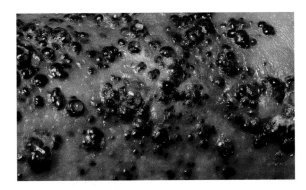

Figure 5.2
Cutaneous melanoma metastases.

to this, the 2-year survival rate for stage IV melanoma was 15–20% and prognostic factors were the site of the metastatic disease and serum lactate dehydrogenase levels. An elevated lactate dehydrogenase is associated with poor prognosis. Patients with cutaneous metastases have better outcomes than those with cerebral metastatic disease.

Numerous trials are under way to investigate immunotherapy and targeted agents for the management of advanced melanoma. The targeted therapies to date have been aimed at inhibiting the BRAF molecular signaling pathway, which is mutated in many melanomas. Vemurafenib is the first BRAF inhibitor to be licensed in the USA and Europe for the treatment of unresectable or metastatic melanomas with a specific mutation (V600E) in the *BRAF* gene. For this patient group, vemurafenib significantly improves progression-free and overall survival rates when compared with conventional dacarbazine chemotherapy. Additional inhibitors that target other mutated pathways in melanoma are in development, including MEK and Kit.

Recent immunomodulatory therapies have also demonstrated survival benefits. Ipilimumab is a monoclonal antibody that blocks a ligand, cytotoxic T lymphocyte antigen 4 (CTLA-4), on cytotoxic T lymphocytes, allowing the cells to continue their cytotoxic action. Survival rates are improved in patients with metastatic melanoma after receiving ipilimumab either as a monotherapy or in combination with dacarbazine. Ipilimumab is licensed in the USA, UK and Europe for the treatment of advanced melanoma. With such rapid advances in this area, there is hope that the management and prognosis of metastatic melanoma will be revolutionized.

Key points – prognosis

- Basal cell carcinoma is a slow-growing tumor that very rarely metastasizes.
- Approximately 3% of extragenital in situ squamous cell carcinoma (SCC) will progress to invasive SCC.
- SCC that is large, undifferentiated, recurrent or at a high-risk location is associated with a poorer prognosis.
- Approximately 5% of lentigo maligna transform into lentigo maligna melanoma.
- The Breslow thickness is the strongest prognostic factor for melanoma.

Key references

Chong K, Daud A, Oritz-Urda S, Arron ST. Cutting edge in medical management of cutaneous oncology. *Semin Cutan Med Surg* 2012;31:140–9.

Edge SB, Byrd DR, Compton CC et al. Melanoma of the skin. In: *AJCC Cancer Staging Handbook*, 7th edn. New York: Springer, 2010:387–415.

Eggermont AM, Robert C. New drugs in melanoma: it's a whole new world. *Eur J Cancer* 2011;47: 2150–7.

Marsden JR, Newton-Bishop JA, Burrows L et al. Revised U.K. guidelines for the management of cutaneous melanoma 2010. *Br J Dermatol* 2010;163:238–56.

Exposure to ultraviolet (UV) radiation is the strongest recognized risk factor for cutaneous malignancy. Therefore, sun-protection strategies are fundamental in the prevention of skin cancer, and sunbeds should be avoided. High-risk individuals require education, self-examination and close observation so that an early diagnosis can be made.

Chemoprophylaxis has a role in very high-risk patients who develop recurrent non-melanoma skin cancer.

Protection from the sun

Taking measures to protect the skin from the sun limits the penetration of UV radiation into the skin, minimizing the risk of photocarcinogenesis, photoimmunosuppression and photo-aging. Protection against UV light involves avoiding the sun, wearing protective clothing and using sunscreens. Individuals, particularly children, should not get sunburn.

Sun avoidance. Exposure to UV irradiation can be significantly reduced by avoiding the midday sun. The intensity of the UV light varies considerably throughout the day, with approximately two-thirds of all UVB and half of UVA radiation reaching the earth between 10 AM and 4 PM. Furthermore, a greater percentage of body surface area is irradiated by sunlight in the middle of the day when the sun is overhead. During this period, 50% of UVB still reaches shaded areas.

Individuals at high risk of skin cancer should limit their lifelong recreational sun exposure. This includes those with fair skin, multiple nevi, freckles, skin that burns in the sun, red or blond hair, and/or a family history of melanoma.

Sunscreens are topically applied lotions or creams that attenuate UV radiation. They can work in two ways:
- reflection of UV light by molecular scattering
- absorption of UV light by the cream and re-emittance as heat.

Sunscreens with a high sun protection factor (SPF) have only been available since the 1980s.

To be effective, a sunscreen must remain on the skin in sufficient quantity throughout the period of sun exposure. Studies on the use of sunscreens by the public show that preparations are generally applied inadequately, with individuals repeatedly using less than the recommended amount. However, when they are used properly, sunscreens appear to be safe and effective.

Sunscreen should be applied 30 minutes before each exposure and reapplied after 2 hours, or after swimming, sweating or toweling off. Used correctly, a tablespoon is required to cover the face and 2 ounces (a shot glass) to cover exposed areas of the body. Patients should also be advised that makeup products containing sunscreen do not provide adequate coverage, particularly as they are rarely used on the ears, neck or chest.

The effectiveness of a sunscreen is primarily assessed by the SPF, a measurement that quantifies the degree of protection provided from the erythemogenic wavelengths, which are primarily UVB. The SPF value is obtained after dividing the minimal erythema dose in sunscreen-protected skin by the minimal erythema dose in non-sunscreen-protected skin.

For non-melanoma skin cancer, the relationship between UVB radiation and photocarcinogenesis is well recognized. However, uncertainty regarding the role of UVA remains, and the UV wavelengths involved in melanoma are unknown. Most sunscreens now offer UVA and UVB protection; a universally standardized measure of UVA protection has yet to be elucidated. The American Academy of Dermatology (AAD) recommends using a sunscreen with both UVA and UVB protection, and with an SPF of 15 or higher. In Australia and New Zealand the recommendation is for a broad-spectrum SPF 30+ sunscreen.

In vitro, sunscreens have been shown to prevent photo-immunosuppression and the formation of UV-radiation-induced pyrimidine dimers and sunburn cells (keratinocytes undergoing apoptosis as a result of UV radiation). Studies have demonstrated that regular application of sunscreen prevents the development of actinic keratoses. Careful regular sunscreen use has also been shown to reduce the occurrence of SCC. One study showed that the regular application of SPF 15+ sunscreen for the first 18 years of life significantly reduced the lifetime risk of non-melanoma skin cancer.

Whether sunscreens can reduce the risk of melanoma has not yet been proven. Epidemiological studies have provided conflicting results and contain many inadequacies. For example, a common bias is seen with individuals who frequently apply sunscreens as they also tend to have a greater degree of sun exposure. It is difficult and probably unethical to perform a reliable study.

Protective clothing offers excellent photoprotection. A given fabric will scatter UVB more than UVA; however, clothing tends to absorb the spectrum of solar irradiation uniformly. The degree of UV protectiveness of a fabric can be expressed as UV protection factor (UPF). UPF is analogous to SPF for sunscreens and is calculated measuring transmission of UVA and UVB through given fabrics with a spectrophotometer. Fabrics with a tight weave, a dark color and a heavy weight are more protective and have a higher UPF. Denim has a UPF of 1700.

Wetness also alters the degree of protection; for example, a white cotton t-shirt provides protection of approximately UPF 6 when dry and UPF 3 when wet.

As individuals are most commonly standing upright when exposed to sunlight, the sites of greatest irradiation include the scalp, face, upper back, forearms and hands. A wide-brimmed hat is particularly protective; wearing a hat with a 10-cm brim has been shown to lower the lifetime rate of skin cancer significantly.

Vitamin D. The skin is the primary source of vitamin D for the body. UVB radiation is required for the production of the vitamin D prohormone within the skin. Vitamin D is essential for bone mineralization and is also important for muscle function. In addition, epidemiological studies have shown an association between vitamin D deficiency and a number of other diseases and cancers. It is therefore inappropriate to rigorously reduce sun exposure in individuals who are not at risk of skin cancer. However, vitamin D supplementation should be considered for those at high risk who take sun-avoidance measures. Studies have identified suboptimal vitamin D levels in melanoma patients, presumably as a result of their behavioral sun-protection measures. There is recent research demonstrating that vitamin D production can be abolished when sunscreen is applied at the recommended thickness.

Skin-cancer prevention campaigns. The combined photoprotective approach of avoiding the sun, wearing appropriate clothing and using regular broad-spectrum high SPF sunscreen is currently the evidence-based recommendation of the AAD. This approach has been shown to reduce the incidence of non-melanoma skin cancer and appears to be reducing the incidence of melanoma.

In Australia, evidence suggests that the incidence of skin cancer is decreasing in people under the age of 50 who have been exposed to long-running sun-protection messages such as the 'slip, slop, slap' (slip on a shirt, slop on sunscreen, slap on a hat) campaign. A similar message has been promoted in the UK since 2003 when the UK Health Departments launched the SunSmart campaign, run by Cancer Research UK. The campaign focuses on the SunSmart message:

• Stay in the shade between 11 AM and 3 PM
• Make sure you never burn
• Always cover up
• Remember to take extra care of children
• Then use factor 15+ sunscreen.

Chemoprophylaxis

Chemoprophylaxis may be suitable and valuable for patients who develop recurrent non-melanoma skin cancer. The administration of systemic retinoids as first-line chemoprophylactic treatment is an area of intensive research. Retinoids exhibit antineoplastic properties and are thought to work by binding nuclear receptors that enhance gene expression for cell differentiation and growth regulation. They tend to be offered to high-risk individuals, such as organ-transplant recipients and patients with xeroderma pigmentosum or basal cell nevus syndrome.

There is evidence that acitretin, 0.3 mg/kg/day, significantly reduces the development of non-melanoma skin cancers in renal transplant recipients who have previously developed SCC or BCC. Continuous treatment is required to maintain the protective effect; the benefit is quickly lost after the retinoid is discontinued.

Key points – prevention

- Protective measures against ultraviolet (UV) radiation involve wearing appropriate clothing, avoiding the sun and using sunscreens.
- Recommended sunscreens have both UVA and UVB protection, with a sun protection factor (SPF) of 15 or greater.
- Regular application of sunscreen in childhood has been shown to reduce the lifetime risk of non-melanoma skin cancer.
- Vitamin D supplementation should be considered in those who rigorously limit sun exposure.
- Oral retinoid prophylaxis can be offered to very-high-risk individuals to reduce the development of non-melanoma skin cancer.

Key references

Australian Cancer Network Melanoma Guidelines Revision Working Party. *Clinical Practice Guidelines for the Management of Melanoma in Australia and New Zealand*. Wellington: Cancer Council Australia and Australian Cancer Network, Sydney and New Zealand Guidelines Group, 2008. Available at www.nhmrc.gov.au/_files_nhmrc/publications/attachments/cp111.pdf, last accessed 19 August 2013.

Bastuji-Garin S, Diepgen TL. Cutaneous malignant melanoma, sun exposure, and sunscreen use: epidemiological evidence. *Br J Dermatol* 2002;146(suppl 61): 24–30.

Faurschou A, Beyer DM, Schmedes A et al. The relation between sunscreen layer thickness and vitamin D production after ultraviolet B exposure: a randomized clinical trial. *Br J Dermatol* 2012;167:391–5.

Kullavanijaya P, Lim HW. Photoprotection. *J Am Acad Dermatol* 2005;52:937–58.

Lim HW, Naylor M, Honigsmann H et al. American Academy of Dermatology Consensus Conference on UVA protection of sunscreens: summary and recommendations. *J Am Acad Dermatol* 2001;44:505–8.

Mahroos MA, Yaar M, Phillips TJ et al. Effect of sunscreen application on UV-induced thymine dimers. *Arch Dermatol* 2002;138:1480–5.

Makin JK, Warne CD, Dobbinson MA et al. Population and age group trends in weekend sun protection and sunburn over two decades of the SunSmart programme in Melbourne, Australia. *Br J Dermatol* 2013;168:154–61.

Rigel DS. Photoprotection: a 21st century perspective. *Br J Dermatol* 2002;146(suppl 61):34–7.

This is a pivotal time in the history of skin cancer and its therapies. The incidence of both non-melanoma skin cancer and melanoma has risen greatly over the past century – more than twentyfold in the case of melanoma – and continues to increase at an alarming rate. Although there is justified concern about the effects of the chemically induced thinning of the ozone layer, the increased numbers of people with skin cancer reflect, in large part, increases in and altered patterns of sun exposure in parts of the population. Changing dress and lifestyles, increased leisure time, the popular convictions that sun exposure is healthy and a tan is attractive, greater longevity and the affordability of distant travel to sunny climes have conspired to put a greater skin surface area at far higher risk from early adulthood into advanced old age.

'Safe sun' campaigns

Only after an unfortunate lag of 30–40 years has research progressively documented the central role of ultraviolet (UV) radiation in skin carcinogenesis. The causal relationship between UV radiation and skin cancer is corroborated by cellular, molecular and animal studies, as well as by epidemiological data. Dissemination of this information has given rise to more widely and effectively used sunscreens and to public health 'safe sun' programs, such as the comprehensive campaign promoted in Australia, where the combination of high isolation, a fair-skinned population and an outdoor lifestyle has resulted in the highest incidence of skin cancer in the world.

Such campaigns offer the possibility of reversing the decades-long trends in morbidity and mortality from non-melanoma skin cancer and melanoma. In Australia, there is evidence to suggest that the incidence of skin cancer decreased in people under the age of 50 who were exposed to long-running sun-protection messages. Thus, it appears that UV radiation, the most prevalent human carcinogen and contributor to more than half of all human malignancies, is on the threshold of simple behavioral control; if adopted widely, conventional sun avoidance and strategies to protect people from the sun are predicted to prevent an estimated 90% of non-melanoma skin cancers and two-thirds of melanomas in the 21st century. It will be fascinating to learn whether humans will exercise this option, for one can enjoy sunshine while being more than 95% protected from unwanted sequelae. This is in contrast to the use of tobacco products, probably the second most prevalent source of carcinogens in modern society.

Novel therapies

'High-tech' approaches to skin-cancer prevention may also shift the present balance between carcinogenic tissue damage and recovery. For example, applying a bacteriophage-derived DNA-repair protein to skin before or soon after sun exposure has already been demonstrated to reduce subsequent photocarcinogenesis. It also appears that the skin's innate protective 'SOS' response to DNA damage can be stimulated by topical application of a DNA fragment that mimics the physiological damage signal, without requiring the otherwise obligatory initial damage. The fragment alters the transcription rate of key genes, increasing both melanogenesis (tanning) and the repair capacity for future UV-induced photoproducts, thus decreasing the risk of skin cancer.

Chemoprevention

The use of a medication to arrest cancer progression in already substantially sun-damage-'initiated' skin is likely to become an important adjunct to the current approach of close observation with biopsy of suspect areas. The first and best-documented chemopreventives are retinoids, compounds derived from vitamin A or their synthetic analogs. Administered either topically or orally, chemopreventive agents – for example, all-*trans*-retinoic acid – can reduce the number of discrete new premalignant and malignant lesions on the skin or oral and respiratory mucosae. Much effort is now being expended to harness this effect while minimizing the potential short- and long-term side effects.

It has also been ascertained that prostaglandin metabolism is elevated in squamous cell carcinoma (SCC) as a result of overexpression of the enzyme cyclooxygenase (COX)-2, which is induced by UV. Orally administered COX-2 inhibitors, now used most commonly to treat arthritis, appear to be promising agents for the prevention of cancers of the skin and intestinal mucosa. Additionally, inhibitors of ornithine decarboxylase, an enzyme required for cellular proliferation, have been shown to prevent both UV- and chemically induced tumors, as have various natural substances found in green tea, grapes and other foodstuffs, at least in animal models.

Biological therapies

Our understanding of the molecular events leading to non-melanoma skin cancer and melanoma has increased greatly in recent years. Particularly well documented are the roles of:

- mutations of the tumor suppressor *P53* gene in SCC
- *PTCH1* or *SMO* mutations in basal cell carcinoma (BCC), resulting in deregulation of basal cell proliferation
- loss of p16INK4a, a protein that inhibits progression through the cell cycle, in melanoma.

In the foreseeable future, our understanding of the complex checks and balances that govern normal skin maintenance, as well as our appreciation of the defining characteristics for malignant versus physiological cell behaviors, may see targeted medical therapy replacing today's surgical procedures. It is already well documented that such medical approaches can eliminate actinic keratoses, the precursors of SCC known to harbor the same p53 mutations as the frankly cancerous lesions. The variety of topical agents now available for actinic keratoses (see Chapter 4) underscore how effective metabolic toxins and immunomodulators have proved to be in the treatment of these lesions. Systemic agents that target the molecular damage in skin cancer, such as vismodegib for BCC or vemurafenib for melanoma, are being rapidly developed as well.

Other therapies eliminate skin cancer by affecting the cutaneous immune response, inducing cytokine synthesis and stimulating lymphocytes to attack the abnormal tumor cells. In the future,

109

targeting formation of new blood vessels, and hence depriving tumors of the nutrients they need, may provide another selective treatment modality. These powerful biological approaches will contribute to our current armamentarium of surgery, radiation and chemotherapy for advanced skin cancer.

Key references

Bissonette R, Bergeron A, Liu Y. Large surface photodynamic therapy with aminolevulinic acid: treatment of actinic keratoses and beyond. *J Drugs Dermatol* 2004;3(suppl 1): S26–31.

Chong K, Daud A, Oritz-Urda S, Arron ST. Cutting edge in medical management of cutaneous oncology. *Semin Cutan Med Surg* 2012;31:140–9.

De Graaf YG, Euvrard S, Bouwes Bavinck JN. Systemic and topical retinoids in the management of skin cancer in organ-transplant recipients. *Dermatol Surg* 2004;30:656–61.

Gilchrest BA. Using DNA damage responses to prevent and treat skin cancers. *J Dermatol* 2004;31: 862–77.

Goukassian DA, Helms E, von Steeg H et al. Topical DNA oligonucleotide therapy reduces UV-induced mutations and photocarcinogenesis in hairless mice. *Proc Natl Acad Sci USA* 2004;101:3 933–8.

Marmur ES, Schmults CD, Goldberg DJ. A review of laser and photodynamic therapy for the treatment of nonmelanoma skin cancer. *Dermatol Surg* 2004;30: 264–71.

Silapunt S, Goldberg LH, Alam M. Topical and light-based treatments for actinic keratoses. *Semin Cutan Med Surg* 2003;22:162–70.

Touma D, Yaar M, Whitehead S et al. A trial of short incubation, broad-area photodynamic therapy for facial actinic keratoses and diffuse photodamage. *Arch Dermatol* 2004;140:33–40.

Yarosh D, Klein J, O'Connor A et al. Effect of topically applied T4 endonuclease V in liposomes in skin cancer in xeroderma pigmentosum: a randomized study. *Lancet* 2001;357:926–69.

Useful resources

UK
British Association of
Dermatologists
Tel: +44 (0)20 7383 0266
admin@bad.org.uk
www.bad.org.uk

British Association of Plastic,
Reconstructive and Aesthetic
Surgeons
Tel: +44 (0)20 7831 5161
secretariat@bapras.org.uk
www.bapras.org.uk

British Skin Foundation
Tel: +44 (0)20 7391 6341
www.britishskinfoundation.org.uk

Cancer Research UK
Tel: +44 (0)20 7242 0200
www.cancerresearchuk.org

Macmillan Cancer Support
Freephone: 0808 808 00 00
www.macmillan.org.uk

Primary Care Dermatology
Society
Tel: +44 (0)1707 226024
pcds@pcds.org.uk
www.pcds.org.uk

SunSmart Campaign
(Cancer Research UK)
www.sunsmart.org.uk

USA
American Academy of
Dermatology
Toll-free: 1 866 503 7546
Tel: +1 847 240 1280
www.aad.org

American College of Mohs
Surgery
Tel: +1 414 347 1103
www.mohscollege.org

American Melanoma Foundation
www.melanomafoundation.org

American Skin Association
Tel: +1 212 889 4858
info@americanskin.org
www.americanskin.org

Skin Cancer Foundation
Tel: +1 212 725 5176
www.skincancer.org

Xeroderma Pigmentosum Society
Tel: +1 518 851 3466
www.xps.org

International

Australasian College of Dermatologists
Tel: +61 (0)2 8741 4101
www.dermcoll.edu.au

Canadian Skin Cancer Foundation
Tel: +1 780 423 2723
www.canadianskincancer
foundation.com

Cancer Council Australia
www.cancer.org.au

Cancer Society of New Zealand
Helpline: 0800 226 237
Tel: +64 (0)4 494 7270
admin@cancersociety.org.nz
www.cancernz.org.nz

DermNet NZ: the dermatology resource (New Zealand)
New Zealand Dermatological Society Incorporated
www.dermnetnz.org

Lentigo Maligna Melanoma: A Sufferer's Tale
Augur Press 2012
www.lentigomalignamelanoma.info

Melanoma Foundation of New Zealand
Toll-free: 0800 463 526
Tel: +64 (0)9 449 2342
admin@melanoma.org.nz
www.melanoma.org.nz

Melanoma International Foundation
Toll-free: 1 866 463 6663
Tel: +1 610 942 3432
contact@melanomainternational.org
www.melanomaintl.org

Nevus Support Australia
Tel: +61 (0)8 8298 3080
michelle@nevussupport.com
www.nevussupport.com

Skin and Cancer Foundation Australia
Tel: +61 (0)2 8833 3000
www.scfa.edu.au

Index

RAS family proteins 18, 24
retinoblastoma 18–19
retinoblastoma protein
  (pRb) 19, 24
retinoids 104–5, 108

'safe sun' campaigns 104,
  107–8
scars, tumors arising in
  54
sebaceous hyperplasia
  47, 48
sebaceous nevus 10, 46
seborrheic keratosis 6,
  33–4
self-examination 76,
  77
senile lentigo 41
sentinel lymph node
  biopsy 90, 97
seven-point checklist,
  melanoma 62
shave biopsy 28
skin types, Fitzpatrick 79
'slip, slop, slap' campaign
  104
SMO mutations 109
solar keratosis see actinic
  keratosis
speckled lentiginous nevus
  39
Spitz nevus 32, 76

squamous cell carcinoma
  (SCC) 6, 7, 50–4
epidemiology 10–13
in situ 50–2, 85–6, 95
invasive 52–4, 86–8, 95–6
pathogenesis 23, 24, 25–6
prevention 103
prognosis 95–6
risk factors 11–13
staging 54, 55
treatment 85–6, 86–8
subungual hematoma 60
subungual malignant
  melanoma 57, 59, 62
sun avoidance 101
sun exposure
  cancer risk 9–10, 11–12,
    14–15
  patterns 25–6
  prevention campaigns
    104, 107–8
  protection from 101–3
sun protection factor (SPF)
  6, 102
sunbed use, excessive 79
sunburn cells 6, 102
sunscreens 101–3
SunSmart campaign 104
surgery 7–8, 71–3
  basal cell carcinoma 82–3
  keratoacanthoma 86
  melanoma 88–9

surgery continued
  squamous cell carcinoma
    85, 87
Sutton's nevus 31–2

topical therapies 69
TP53 (P53) gene 19, 23,
  25, 109
treatments 69–74
tumor suppressor genes
  18–19

ultraviolet protection
  factor (UPF) 6, 103
ultraviolet (UV) radiation 6
  cancer risk 9–10, 11–12, 14
  mechanism of
    carcinogenesis 20–2
  patterns of exposure 25–6
  protection from 101–3
  'safe sun' campaigns 104,
    107–8
  substantial exposure,
    management 78–9

vemurafenib 99, 109
verrucous carcinoma 52–3
viral infections 25
vismodegib 84, 109
vitamin D 7, 103–4

xeroderma pigmentosum 6,
  23, 78, 105

Your Aha! Moment?

A moment of sudden realization, inspiration, insight, recognition or comprehension

Did you have one when reading this text? That is our aim at *Fast Facts*, but we don't want you to keep it to yourself. Share your Aha! Moments and read others at:

www.fastfacts.com/fast-facts/Skin-Cancer-2nd-edn

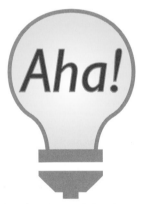

And if you found this book useful, please consider sharing it with your colleagues or students. A book recommendation from someone you work with is often the best kind, so send this title on a journey around your clinic or department and help us on our mission **to promote health, effectively.**